UNDERSTANDING 12-LEAD EKGs

A PRACTICAL APPROACH

Brenda Beasley
BS, RN, EMT-Paramedic

Michael West
MS, RN, EMT-Paramedic

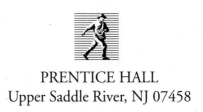

PRENTICE HALL
Upper Saddle River, NJ 07458

Library of Congress Cataloging-in-Publication Data

Beasley, Brenda M.
  Understanding 12-lead EKGs : a practical approach / Brenda
Beasley, Mike West.
      p.   cm.
  Companion v. to: Understanding EKGs. c1999.
  Includes index.
  ISBN 0-13-027281-7 (alk. paper)
  1. Electrocardiography.   I. West, Mike, (date)   II.
  Beasley, Brenda M. Understanding EKGs.   III. Title.
      [DNLM: 1. Electrocardiography.   2. Myocardial
      Infarction—diagnosis. WG 140 B3676ua 2000]
  RC683.5.E5 B374   2000
  616.1'207547—dc21
                                                00-058902

Publisher: Julie Alexander
Executive Editor: Greg Vis
Acquisitions Editor: Katrin Beacom
**Director of Production
  and Manufacturing:** Bruce Johnson
Managing Production Editor: Patrick Walsh
Production Editor: Stephanie Landis, North Market Street Graphics
Production Liaison: Larry Hayden IV
Manufacturing Manager: Ilene Sanford
Creative Director: Marianne Frasco
Cover Image: "Angioplasty, ©2000 Cynthia Turner
Cover Design Coordinator: Maria Guglielmo
Marketing Director: Leslie Cavaliere
Marketing Manager: Tiffany Price
Composition: North Market Street Graphics
Printing and Binding: Press of Ohio

Prentice-Hall International (UK) Limited, *London*
Prentice-Hall of Australia Pty. Limited, *Sydney*
Prentice-Hall Canada Inc., *Toronto*
Prentice-Hall Hispanoamericana, S.A., *Mexico*
Prentice-Hall of India Private Limited, *New Delhi*
Prentice-Hall of Japan, Inc., *Tokyo*
Prentice-Hall Singapore Pte. Ltd.
Editora Prentice-Hall do Brasil, Ltda., *Rio de Janeiro*

10 9 8 7 6 5 4 3 2 1
ISBN 0-13-027281-7

DEDICATION

This book is dedicated to the memory of a man who was a consummate EMS professional, a wonderful human being, and a good friend,

Larry G. Gosdin Sr.

The very thought of Larry brings to mind one of my favorite sayings:

Some people come into our lives and quietly go; others stay awhile, leave footprints on our hearts, and we are never the same.

We'll all miss you, my friend . . . rest well, until we meet again.

B.M.B.

CONTENTS

FOREWORD

The value of over 30 years of combined EMS educational experience enables Brenda Beasley and Michael West to bring a unique and insightful approach to the topic of 12-lead EKGs and their interpretation. The authors have presented a complex, yet vitally important subject in a comprehensive, straightforward, and easy-to-understand format.

The text serves a wide audience of health care providers, including pre-hospital providers, nurses, physician assistants, respiratory therapists, and anyone requiring a thorough understanding of electrocardiography. I believe that this book fills a void in the subject matter of EKG interpretation. It demonstrates the ability to educate medical personnel who are new to the subject matter while providing a review to those who are more experienced.

Using a reader-friendly writing style, the authors create a text that begins with the basics of EKG interpretation, then introduces a building-block approach to a more detailed discussion of this topic. Many illustrations, tables, and graphs are used to help highlight the important issues of each topic. Also, the reader will find the review questions at the end of each chapter useful in helping to solidify knowledge of salient issues.

Ms. Beasley has played a vital role in EMS education throughout the state of Alabama. She has made a difference in the lives of many people as well as influenced many career decisions. It was her commitment to education in and excitement about emergency medicine that was a significant factor in my choice of medicine as a career and, later, emergency medicine as a profession. The nursing background of both Ms. Beasley and Mr. West, and their experience as EMS educators, give them the wisdom to continue their roles of educating and influencing others through this text.

The importance of communicating and understanding EKG changes between all medical personnel cannot be overemphasized. As an emergency medicine physician, I congratulate both Ms. Beasley and Mr. West on a book that provides common ground between physicians, nurses, and pre-hospital personnel.

Benjamin J. Camp, MD

AUTHOR ACKNOWLEDGMENTS

This textbook was developed and created from our collective experiences in EMS education as well as in the clinical practice of emergency medicine. In order to develop a comprehensive, yet logical 12-lead EKG text, we called on the assistance and advice of numerous friends and colleagues. We wish to recognize the following individuals who were instrumental, each in his or her own unique way, in making this textbook a reality. We offer our sincere appreciation to:

The awesome team at Brady! The support of Julie Alexander has been unwavering and much appreciated. Judy Streger has been our champion, our most ardent supporter, and our "guardian angel" throughout the first nine months of this project. Where Judy left off, Katrin Beacom stepped in and skillfully guided us through the completion of the project. Jeanne Molenaar has consistently been involved with every phase of the review process and has done a remarkable job. A very special thank you to Tiffany Price and her team for lending their considerable marketing expertise to us during the promotion of this book as well as the companion book. The numerous demands of production have been in the very competent and efficient hands of Patrick Walsh, production manager, and Larry Hayden, production liaison. Stephanie Landis and Jill Lynch at North Market Street Graphics have been wonderful to work with and have guided us well through this stage of the process.

Our informal reviewer, Dr. Willis D. Israel, whose review of this text has been another example of his positive influence on EMS education throughout many years. Thank you, Dr. I.!

Dr. Ben Camp, for writing the foreword for this book as well as for lending his advice and expertise to us throughout the entire project.

Our expert reviewers, Jarrod Taylor, Dr. Ben Camp, Judith Ruple, Chuck Carter, John Beckman, Marilyn Ermish, and Jim Williams, who have consistently provided excellent suggestions and ideas for improving the text.

In addition, we gratefully acknowledge the following employees of Athens-Limestone Hospital Emergency Department and Emergency Medical Services for all their contributions to the development of this manuscript: Rick Solís, Andy Jackson, Shane Jackson, Eddie West, Ginger West, Dannie Stinnett, Jeff Crawford, Jarrod Taylor, Bret McGill, Chuck Godwin, J. Brett Kinzer, and Jeff Williams. A special thanks to all the ALH employees who gathered hundreds of 12-lead strips for us!

And, last but not least, we gratefully acknowledge our families, friends, and colleagues for their support, encouragement, and acceptance of our long absences during the development of this text. Without the strength and love we received from each of you, this task would have not been possible. Thank you so much.

PREFACE

Our purpose in writing this book was to create a learning resource that is reader-friendly, yet comprehensive in its approach to the interpretation of the 12-lead electrocardiogram. This text serves as a companion text to *Understanding EKGs: A Practical Approach.*

This book consists of 18 chapters that are designed to provide the user with a practical approach to the skill of 12-lead EKG interpretation. The goal of this text is to focus on providing a useful and understandable tool for the health care provider in his/her provision of optimum patient care.

It has been our intent that the presentation of the material be accomplished in a logical order. In order to afford the student the opportunity to work in a reasonable order through the technical information, the material is presented in such a manner as to achieve understanding of each chapter prior to proceeding to the next chapter. The content is presented in short, succinct chapters in order to facilitate comprehension of each concept in a "building block" format. At the end of each chapter, we have included a section of multiple choice questions to be used as self-assessment and review.

A thorough knowledge of basic EKG interpretation is an essential prerequisite to understanding 12-lead EKG interpretation. With this thought in mind, we began this book with a series of chapters reviewing basic dysrhythmia interpretation. This book includes rhythm strip examples within each applicable chapter, as well as an entire chapter devoted to 12-lead EKG review strips. In addition, there are chapters devoted to cardiovascular pharmacology and therapeutic modalities.

Since the late 1980s, the use of thrombolytics in the treatment of acute myocardial infarctions has become an ever expanding, dynamic component of the health care professions. As a direct result of this, more and more health care providers are required to interpret, understand, and apply their knowledge of 12-lead EKGs in the clinical setting.

We sincerely hope that this logical, yet comprehensive approach to 12-lead EKG interpretation will furnish the student, as well as other health care providers, with a substantial foundation for the interpretation and understanding of electrocardiology. Ultimately, it is our wish that your future patients will benefit from the knowledge that you attain from this text.

1

THE ANATOMY OF THE HEART (STRUCTURE)

Objectives

Upon completion of this chapter, the student will be able to:

1. Identify the location, shape, and size of the heart
2. Describe the chambers of the heart:
   a. Atria
   b. Ventricles
3. Name and locate the layers of the heart
4. Name and locate the valves of the heart
5. Describe the structure and function of the blood vessels:
   a. Arteries
   b. Veins
   c. Capillaries

It is our belief that in order to properly master the art of 12-lead EKG interpretation, you must first have a thorough understanding of the structure of the heart. Therefore, this chapter provides you with a foundation upon which to review the fundamental knowledge of basic dysrhythmia interpretation. The focus of this chapter will thus be to provide you with a simple yet comprehensive reassessment of cardiac anatomy. After you have reviewed the basic cardiac anatomy (structure), you will be prepared to move into the next chapter, which reexamines the basic physiology (function) of the heart.

ANATOMY OF THE HEART

As you will learn, the heart is a muscle. Although we don't think of exercising our heart muscle when we go to the gym, the fact is that your heart muscle (**myocardium**) is constantly in the "exercise mode." At times of rest, the exercise is more sedate. Think however, of the vigor with which your heart muscle must exercise when you walk (or run) up six flights of stairs! Now, as you feel your heart pumping, you can easily understand that your heart muscle is indeed exercising!

We often hear the heart referred to as a "two-sided pump," and this analogy works well in our understanding of the basics of cardiac anatomy. Indeed, we can visualize this pump as having a right side and a left side. On each side of the pump, there is an upper chamber that is referred to as the atrium (plural: **atria**) and a lower chamber known as the ventricle. There are a total of four hollow chambers in the normal heart. Again, the two upper chambers of the heart are called atria, while the two lower chambers are called ventricles.

The upper chambers are separated by the interatrial septum, and the lower chambers are separated by the interventricular septum. Externally, the atrioventricular groove divides the atria from the ventricles. The anterior and posterior interventricular grooves separate the ventricles externally. The muscle fibers of the ventricles are continuous, as are the atrial muscle fibers.

The two upper chambers of the heart are located at the base, or top, of the heart, while the lower chambers are located at the bottom, or apex, of the heart. The upper chambers of the heart are thin-walled and receive blood as it returns to the heart. The lower chambers of the heart have thicker walls and pump blood away from the heart, throughout the systemic circulation (Fig. 1-1).

LOCATION, SIZE, AND SHAPE OF THE HEART

It is important for you to understand the location of the heart in that the effectiveness of one of our most basic, yet most important skills—namely cardiopulmonary resuscitation (CPR)—depends upon the reasonable knowledge

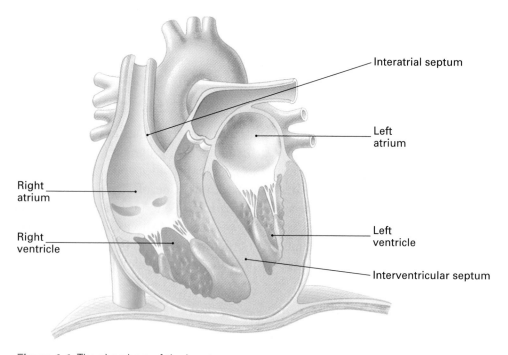

Figure 1-1 The chambers of the heart.

of this position. The proper placement of electrodes to record either a 3-lead or 12-lead electrocardiogram depends upon the proper understanding of the location of the heart.

The central section of the thorax (chest cavity) is called the mediastinum. It is in this area where the heart is housed, lying in front of the spinal column, behind the sternum, and between the lungs (see Fig. 1-2). When thinking of the heart muscle in terms of its mass, one should realize that two-thirds of the heart muscle lies to the left of the midline. The apex of the heart lies just above the diaphragm, while the base of the heart lies at approximately the level of the third rib.

The exact size of the heart varies somewhat among individuals, but on average it is approximately 5 inches or 10–12 centimeters in length and 3 inches or 9 centimeters wide. The shape of the heart is somewhat conelike. It is appropriate to visualize the heart as approximately the size of its owner's closed fist.

LAYERS OF THE HEART

The Pericardium

Surrounding the heart is a closed, two-layered sac referred to as the pericardium, also known as the pericardial sac. In direct contact with the pleura is the outer layer, or the parietal pericardium. This layer consists of tough, nonelastic fibrous connective tissue and serves to prevent overdistension of the heart. The thin, serous inner layer of the pericardium is called the visceral pericardium and is contiguous with the epicardium, which surrounds the heart. A space filled with a scant amount of fluid (approximately 10 cc)

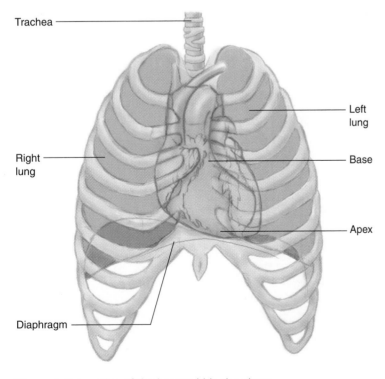

Trachea

Left lung

Right lung

Base

Apex

Diaphragm

Figure 1-2 Location of the heart within the chest.

separates the two pericardial layers. This fluid helps to reduce friction as the heart moves within the pericardial sac by acting as a lubricant.

An inflammation of the serous pericardium is called pericarditis. Although the cause of this disease is frequently unknown, it may result from infection or disease of the connective tissue. This disease can cause severe pain, which may be confused with the pain of myocardial infarction. This can make physical assessment of the cardiac patient a real challenge for the clinician.

The Heart Wall

Three layers of tissue compose the heart wall (see Fig. 1-3). This specialized cardiac muscle tissue is unique to the heart. The epicardium is the smooth outer surface of the heart. The thick middle layer of the heart, called the myocardium, is the thickest of the three layers of the heart wall. The myocardium is composed primarily of cardiac muscle cells and is responsible for the heart's ability to contract. The innermost layer, the endocardium, is composed of thin connective tissue. This smooth inner surface of the heart and heart valves allows blood to flow more easily throughout the heart.

VALVES OF THE HEART

The four valves of the heart allow blood to flow in only one direction. There are two sets of valves, called the atrioventricular valves and the semilunar valves.

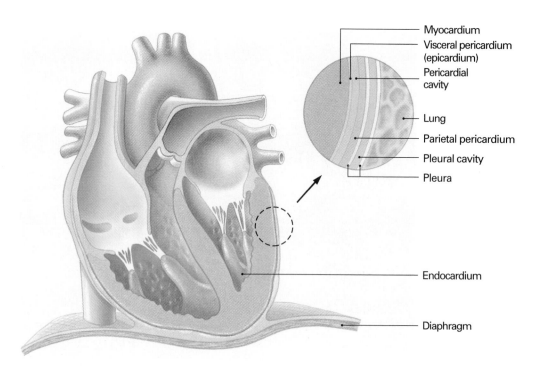

Figure 1-3 Layers of the heart.

The Atrioventricular Valves

As indicated by their name, the atrioventricular valves are located between the atria and the ventricles. These valves allow blood to flow from the atria into the ventricles. They are also effective in preventing blood from flowing backward from the ventricles into the atria.

The tricuspid valve is named for its three cusps and is located between the right atrium and the right ventricle. Free edges of each of the three cusps extend into the ventricles, where they attach to the chordae tendineae. The chordae tendineae are fine cords of dense connective tissue that attach to papillary muscles in the walls of the ventricles. The chordae tendineae and papillary muscles work in concert to prevent the cusps from fluttering back into the atrium and causing disruption of blood flow through the heart.

The mitral (or bicuspid) valve is similar in structure to the tricuspid valve, but has only two cusps. The mitral valve is located between the left atrium and the left ventricle.

The Semilunar Valves

In much the same manner as the atrioventricular valves prevent backflow of blood into the atria, the semilunar valves serve to prevent backflow of blood into the ventricles. Each semilunar valve contains three semilunar (or moon-shaped) cusps. The semilunar valves are the pulmonic and aortic valves. The semilunar valve located between the right ventricle and the pulmonary artery is called the pulmonic valve. The semilunar valve located between the left ventricle and the trunk of the aorta is known as the aortic valve.

Changes in chamber pressure govern the opening and closing of the heart valves. During ventricular systole (contraction of the ventricles), the atrioventricular valves close and the semilunar valves open. During ventricular diastole (relaxation of the ventricles), the aortic and pulmonic valves are closed and the mitral and tricuspid valves are open. Passive filling of the coronary arteries occurs during ventricular diastole.

ARTERIES, VEINS, AND CAPILLARIES

Since we tend to refer to the heart as the body's pump, we can similarly consider the vasculature, or blood vessels, as the container for the fluid (blood). When considering the purpose of this text, it is appropriate to discuss three commonly accepted groups of blood vessels: arteries, veins, and capillaries.

Arteries

Arteries, by virtue of their primary function, are relatively thick-walled and muscular. These blood vessels function under high pressure in order to convey blood from the heart out to the rest of the body. Since one definition of the prefix *a* is *away from,* a helpful hint is to remember that the word *artery* also begins with the letter *a;* thus arteries carry blood **away from** the heart. Larger arterial blood vessels are called arteries; these vessels branch off into smaller blood vessels known as arterioles. Arteries, with the exception of the pulmonary and umbilical arteries, carry oxygenated blood.

Arteries also operate in the regulation of blood pressure through functional changes in peripheral vascular resistance (the amount of opposition to blood flow offered by the arterioles). Arterial walls consist of three distinct layers including the intima, media, and adventitia (see Table 1-1 and Fig. 1-4). These layers are also called tunics (coats or coverings). The tunica intima is the innermost layer and consists of endothelium and an inner elastic membrane. This inner elastic membrane separates the intimal layer from the next layer, the tunica media. The tunica media is the middle layer and consists of smooth muscle cells. It is in this middle layer where the blood flow through the vessel is regulated by constriction or dilation. Vasoconstriction, or a decrease in the diameter of the blood vessel, produces a decrease in blood flow. In contrast, vasodilation, or an increase in the diameter of the blood vessel, produces an increase in blood flow. The tunica adventitia, or outermost layer, is composed of various connective tissues.

Other structures of importance in this discussion are the coronary arteries and the coronary sinus. The right and left coronary arteries arise from the aorta and function to carry oxygenated blood throughout the myocardium. The coronary sinus is a short trunk that serves to receive deoxygenated blood from the veins of the myocardium. This trunk empties into the right atrium.

Veins

Veins are defined as blood vessels that carry blood back to the heart. Veins branch off into smaller vessels known as venules. With the exception of venules, veins are structurally similar to arteries in that they also have three layers. Unlike arteries, however, veins operate under low pressure, are relatively thin-walled, and contain one-way valves. With the exception of the pulmonary vein, the veins convey deoxygenated blood. The larger veins of the body ultimately empty into the two largest veins, the superior

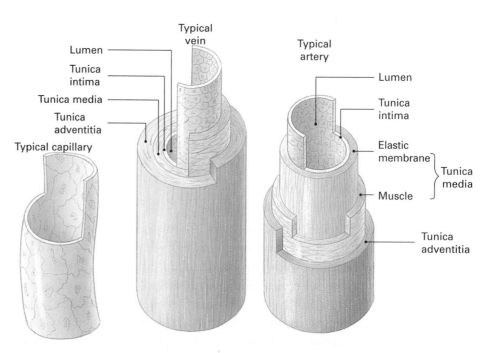

Figure 1-4 Arterial wall layers.

TABLE 1-1 ARTERIAL WALL LAYERS

Name	Layer	Tissue Type
Tunica intima	Innermost	Connective and elastic
Tunica media	Middle	Smooth muscle, elastic, and collagen
Tunica adventitia	Outermost	Connective

vena cava and the inferior vena cava, which empty deoxygenated blood into the heart's right atrium. The superior vena cava drains blood from the head and neck, while the inferior vena cava collects blood from the rest of the body.

Capillaries

Capillaries are tiny blood vessels whose walls are the thinnest of those of all blood vessels. In the human body, there is a greater number of capillaries than of any other type of blood vessel. In fact, capillaries are so tiny that red blood cells must "march through" in single file. From the arterioles, blood flows into the capillaries, where the vast majority of gas exchange occurs.

In summary, arterioles transport oxygenated blood into the capillaries. Capillaries allow for the exchange of oxygen, nutrients, and waste products between the blood and body tissues and are viewed as connectors between arteries and veins. The smallest of the veins—the venules—receive the deoxygenated blood, which travels back to the heart via the venous system.

REVIEW QUESTIONS: CHAPTER 1

1. When reviewing the layers of the heart, you will recall that the fibrous sac covering the heart, which is in contact with the pleura, is called the:

   a. Epicardium

   b. Myocardium

   c. Pericardium

   d. Endocardium

2. The heart chamber with the thickest myocardium is the:

   a. Right ventricle

   b. Left ventricle

3. The pulmonic and aortic valves are open during:

   a. Systole

   b. Diastole

4. The large blood vessel that returns unoxygenated blood from the head and neck to the right atrium is called the:

a. Jugular vein

b. Carotid artery

c. Superior vena cava

d. Inferior vena cava

5. The innermost layer of the arterial wall is called the:

   a. Tunica intima

   b. Tunica media

   c. Myocardium

   d. Tunica adventitia

6. The most numerous blood vessels in the body are the:

   a. Arteries

   b. Capillaries

   c. Venules

   d. Veins

7. Blood flow between the heart and lungs comprises the:

   a. Systemic circulation

   b. Venous circulation

   c. Myocardial circulation

   d. Pulmonary circulation

8. Blood vessels that function under high pressure in order to convey blood from the heart out to the rest of the body are known as the:

   a. Venules

   b. Veins

   c. Arteries

   d. Capillaries

9. The blood vessel that returns unoxygenated blood from the myocardium to the right atrium is called the great cardiac vein or the:

   a. Jugular vein

   b. Carotid artery

   c. Coronary sinus

   d. Inferior vena cava

10. _____ _____ are fine cords of dense connective tissue that attach to papillary muscles in the walls of the ventricles.

    a. Coronary arteries

    b. Coronary sinuses

    c. Chordae tendineae

    d. Purkinje fibers

2

CARDIOVASCULAR PHYSIOLOGY (FUNCTION)

Objectives

Upon completion of this chapter, the student will be able to:

1. Describe the sequence of blood flow through the heart
2. Describe the cardiac cycle, including:
   a. Definition
   b. Systole
   c. Diastole
3. Discuss the term *stroke volume*
4. Discuss cardiac output, preload, Starling's Law, and afterload
5. Describe the autonomic nervous system

Now that we have dealt with the review of the structure of the heart, we will address the basic function (or physiology) of the cardiovascular system. The focus of this chapter will be on providing you with an uncomplicated yet inclusive review of cardiac physiology. After you have mastered the knowledge of basic cardiac physiology (function), you will be prepared to move into the next chapter, which addresses the basic electrophysiology of the heart.

Note:

Now is the perfect time to look back at the review questions from Chapter 1, then proceed on through the objectives and contents of this chapter.

Blood Flow through the Heart

The path of blood flow through the heart is our first consideration in reviewing the physiology of circulation. Imagine that the right atrium is a receptacle that functions, in part, to receive unoxygenated blood from the head, neck, and trunk. In order to simplify the route of circulation, the learner may choose to divide this concept into three components.

The first component consists of blood flow through the right heart, which proceeds as follows:

Unoxygenated blood flows from the inferior and superior venae cavae into the:

Right atrium	Through the tricuspid valve	Into the right ventricle	Through the pulmonic valve

The second component of blood flow through the pulmonary circulation continues when the blood travels from the pulmonic valve into the:

Pulmonary arteries	Into the lungs	Through the pulmonary alveolar-capillary network	Into the pulmonary veins

The third and final component of blood flow through the pulmonary circulation continues when the blood travels from the pulmonary veins into the:

Left atrium	Through the mitral valve	Into the left ventricles	Through the aortic valve and out to the rest of the body

It should be noted that the freshly oxygenated blood traveling through the aortic valve also enters into the coronary arteries in order to accomplish myocardial oxygenation. The vital function of gas exchange occurs in the second or middle component of pulmonary circulation, when carbon dioxide is exchanged for oxygen in the pulmonary alveolar-capillary network.

Cardiac Cycle

The heart functions as a unit in that both atria contract simultaneously, then both ventricles contract (see Fig. 2-1). When the atria contract, the ventricles are filled to their limits. Blood is ejected into both the pulmonary and systemic circulations when the simultaneous contraction of the ventricles occurs. At the time of ventricular contraction, the mitral and tricuspid valves are closed by the pressure of the contraction and the pull of the papillary muscles, while the pulmonic and aortic valves are opened. The *cardiac cycle* represents the actual time sequence between ventricular contraction and ventricular relaxation.

Systole, also referred to as **ventricular systole,** is consistent with the simultaneous contraction of the ventricles, while *diastole* is synonymous with **ventricular relaxation.** The ventricles fill passively with approxi-

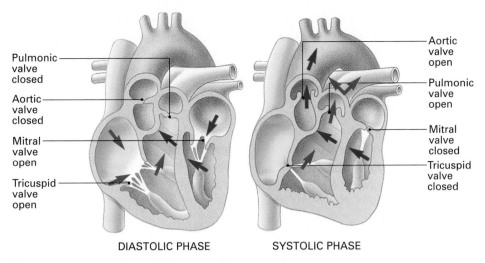

Figure 2-1 Relation of blood flow to cardiac contraction.

mately 70% of the blood that has collected in the atria during ventricular diastole. Then the active contraction of the atria propels the remaining 30% of the blood into the ventricles. Atrial contraction represents only a minimal role in filling; consequently, even if the atria do not contract effectively, ventricular filling still ensues. During periods of ventricular relaxation, cardiac filling and coronary perfusion occur passively.

One cardiac cycle occurs every 0.8 second. Systole lasts about 0.28 second, while diastole lasts about 0.52 second. Thus, the period of diastole is substantially longer than the period of systole.

STROKE VOLUME

Stroke volume may be defined as the volume of blood pumped out of one ventricle of the heart in a single beat or contraction. Stroke volume is estimated at approximately 70 cubic centimeters per beat. The number of contractions, or beats per minute, is known as the heart rate. The normal heart rate is 60 to 100 beats per minute (BPM).

CARDIAC OUTPUT

Cardiac output is the amount of blood pumped by the left ventricle in 1 minute. The output of the right ventricle is normally considered to be equal to that of the left, since these two chambers contract simultaneously. By remembering the following formula, we can determine the cardiac output:

Cardiac output (CO) =	Stroke volume (SV) × Heart rate (HR)

Consequently, if a patient has a heart rate of 80 beats per minute and a stroke volume of 70 cubic centimeters per beat, the resulting cardiac output will be approximately 5,600 cubic centimeters per minute (or 5.6 l/min). When, for a variety of reasons, the patient's cardiac output is outside the normal range, the heart will try to balance it by changes in either the stroke volume or the heart rate. Inadequate cardiac output may be indicated by a combination of any of the following signs and symptoms: shortness of breath, dizziness, decreased blood pressure, chest pains, and cool and clammy skin.

Commonly called **end-diastolic pressure,** *preload* is the pressure in the ventricles at the end of diastole. *Afterload* is the resistance against which the heart must pump. This pressure also affects stroke volume and cardiac output.

When the volume of blood in the ventricles is increased, stretching the ventricular myocardial fibers and consequently causing a more forceful contraction, a concept known as *Starling's Law of the heart* is the result. This concept is a law of physiology that basically states that the more the myocardial fibers are stretched—up to a certain point—the more forceful the subsequent contraction will be. Thus we can assume that if the volume of blood filling the ventricle increases significantly, so will the force of the cardiac contraction. This law can be thought of as analogous to the stretching of a rubber band (the farther you stretch a rubber band, the harder it snaps back to its original size).

The amount of opposition to blood flow offered by the arterioles is known as the peripheral (or systemic) vascular resistance. If the peripheral vascular resistance remains uniform, a patient's blood pressure may increase or decrease if the cardiac output changes significantly. Vasoconstriction and vasodilation determine peripheral vascular resistance (PVR). Blood pressure is subject to change if the cardiac output or peripheral vascular resistance changes. Therefore it may be helpful to remember the following formula:

Blood pressure (BP) =	Cardiac output (CO) × Peripheral vascular resistance (PVR)

AUTONOMIC NERVOUS SYSTEM

The autonomic nervous system regulates functions of the body that are involuntary or are not under conscious control. Thus, we do not have to consciously think about our heartbeat or about regulating our blood pressure. Heart rate and blood pressure are regulated by this component of the nervous system (see Fig. 2-2).

There are two major divisions of the autonomic nervous system; the sympathetic nervous system and the parasympathetic nervous system. The majority of organs in the body are innervated by both systems. It is important to note that blood vessels are only innervated by the sympathetic nervous system. The sympathetic nervous system is responsible for preparation of the body for physical activity ("fight or flight"), and the parasympathetic nervous system regulates the calmer ("rest and digest") functions of our existence.

RECEPTORS AND NEUROTRANSMITTERS

Nerve endings of the sympathetic nervous system and the parasympathetic nervous system secrete neurotransmitters. The sympathetic nervous system

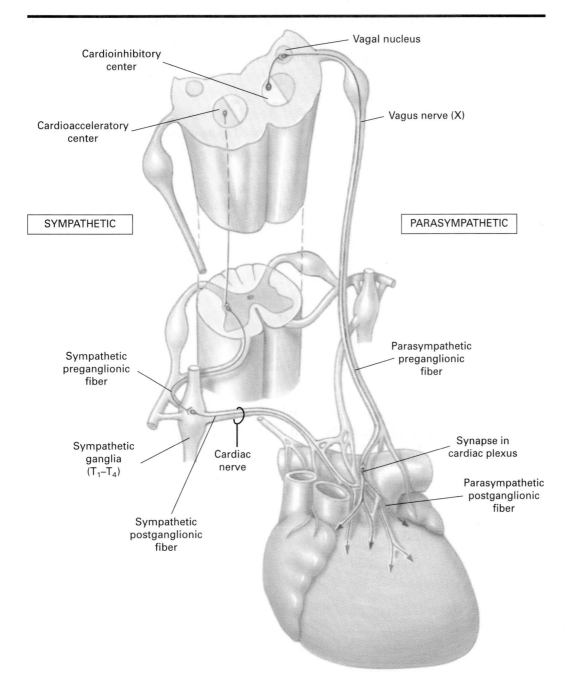

Figure 2-2 Nervous control of the heart.

has two types of receptor fibers at the nerve endings: the alpha and beta receptors. The chemical neurotransmitter for the sympathetic nervous system is norepinephrine. The nerve endings of the sympathetic nervous system are called *adrenergic*. When norepinephrine is released, an increase in heart rate, the contractile force of cardiac fibers, and vasoconstriction will result.

The chemical neurotransmitter for the parasympathetic nervous system is acetylcholine, and the nerve endings are known as *cholinergic*. When acetylcholine is released, the heart rate slows, as do atrioventricular conduction rates. With the exception of capillaries, all of the body's blood vessels have alpha-adrenergic receptors, while the heart and lungs have beta-adrenergic receptors. For further details regarding receptors and neurotransmitters, refer to Chapter 2 of *Understanding EKGs: A Practical Approach,* the companion book to this text.

REVIEW QUESTIONS: CHAPTER 2

1. The left side of the heart is referred to as a low-pressure pump.

   a. True

   b. False

2. The major blood vessel that receives blood from the head and upper extremities and transports it to the heart is the:

   a. Aorta

   b. Superior vena cava

   c. Inferior vena cava

   d. Pulmonary artery

3. The course of blood flow through the heart and lungs is referred to as _____ circulation.

   a. Aortic

   b. Pulmonary

   c. Systemic

   d. Collateral

4. Cardiac output is a factor of:

   a. Cardiac rate

   b. Stroke volume

   c. Partial vascular resistance

   d. a and b

5. The chief chemical neurotransmitter for the parasympathetic nervous system is:

   a. Acetylcholine

   b. Norepinephrine

   c. Epinephrine

   d. Atropine

6. The heart has _____ chambers.

   a. 2

   b. 3

   c. 4

   d. 6

7. The chief chemical neurotransmitter for the sympathetic nervous system is:

   a. Acetylcholine

    b. Norepinephrine

    c. Ephedrine

    d. Atropine

8. Unoxygenated blood flows from the inferior and superior venae cavae into the:

    a. Left atrium

    b. Left ventricle

    c. Right ventricle

    d. Right atrium

9. One cardiac cycle occurs every:

    a. 0.8 second

    b. 0.5 second

    c. 0.52 second

    d. 1.2 seconds

10. With the exception of _____, all of the body's blood vessels have alpha-adrenergic receptors, while the heart and lungs have beta-adrenergic receptors.

    a. Arterioles

    b. Capillaries

    c. Venules

    d. Aorta

3

BASIC ELECTROPHYSIOLOGY

Objectives

Upon completion of this chapter, the student will be able to:

1. State the two basic myocardial cell groups
2. Describe the function of each myocardial cell group
3. Discuss the four primary properties of cardiac cells
4. List the three major electrolytes that affect cardiac function
5. Describe the movement of ions across cell membranes
6. Describe cardiac depolarization
7. Describe cardiac repolarization
8. Define *refractory period*
9. Describe the absolute refractory period
10. Describe the relative refractory period

Although the in-depth study of cardiac electrophysiology can be quite complicated and baffling to the novice student, the intent of this text is to concentrate on a review of the **basics** of dysrhythmia interpretation. Thus this discussion of electrophysiology will center on rudimentary, but very important, concepts.

In our discussion of cardiac anatomy in Chapter 1, we established the fact that the heart is indeed a very unique and distinctive organ, unlike any other organ in the human body. The heart is composed of cardiac muscle, which is made up of thousands of myocardial cells. For purposes of discussion, we will consider that there are two basic myocardial cell groups: the myocardial working cells and the specialized pacemaker cells of the electrical conduction system.

Basic Cell Groups

The Myocardial Working Cells

The myocardial working cells are responsible for generating the physical contraction of the heart muscle. The muscular layer of the wall of the atria, as well as the thicker muscular layer of the ventricular walls, are constructed of myocardial working cells. Myocardial working cells are permeated by contractile filaments, which, when electrically stimulated, produce myocardial contraction. Thus, the primary functions of the myocardial working cells include both contraction and relaxation.

It should be noted that this physical contraction of myocardial tissue actually generates blood flow; however, organized electrical activity is required in order to produce the physical contraction. As the myocardial tissue contracts, the size of the atria and ventricles decreases, producing the ejection of blood from the chambers.

The Specialized Pacemaker Cells

Unlike the myocardial working cells, the specialized pacemaker cells of the electrical conduction system do not contain contractile filaments and thus do not have the ability to contract. Rather, this specialized group of cells is responsible for controlling the rate and rhythm of the heart by coordinating regular depolarization (see the section on cardiac depolarization later in this chapter). These cells are found in the electrical conduction system of the heart. Thus the generation and conduction of electrical impulses are the primary functions of the specialized myocardial pacemaker cells.

Cardiac muscle cells have the ability to contract in response to thermal, chemical, electrical, or mechanical stimuli. All atrial muscle cells contract simultaneously; comparably, all ventricular muscle cells contract together.

The term *threshold* refers to the point at which a stimulus will produce a cell response. When a stimulus is strong enough for cardiac cells to reach threshold, all cells will respond to the stimulus and will thus contract. This is known as the *all or none phenomenon* of cardiac muscle cells; that is, either all cells will respond or none will respond. Hence, cardiac muscle functions on an "all or none" principle.

Primary Cardiac Cell Characteristics

Cardiac cells possess four primary cell characteristics (see Table 3-1). These properties are excitability (or irritability), conductivity, contractility (or rhythmicity), and automaticity. Only one of these characteristics—contractility—is considered a mechanical function of the heart. The other three characteristics—automaticity, excitability, and conductivity—are electrical functions of the heart.

Automaticity is the ability of cardiac pacemaker cells to spontaneously generate their own electrical impulses without external (or nervous) stimu-

TABLE 3-1 PRIMARY CARDIAC CELL CHARACTERISTICS		
Characteristic	Location	Function
Automaticity	SA node, AV junction, Purkinje network fibers	Electrical
Excitability	All cardiac cells	Electrical
Conductivity	All cardiac cells	Electrical
Contractility	Myocardial muscle cells	Mechanical

lation. This intrinsic spontaneous depolarization frequency produces contraction of myocardial muscle cells. This characteristic is specific to the pacemaker cell sites of the electrical conduction system—that is, the sinoatrial (SA) node, the atrioventricular (AV) junction, and the Purkinje network fibers.

Excitability is the ability of cardiac cells to respond to an electrical stimulus. This characteristic is shared by all cardiac cells and is also referred to as *irritability*. A weaker stimulus is required to cause a contraction when a cardiac cell is highly irritable.

Conductivity is the ability of cardiac cells to receive an electrical stimulus and then to transmit the stimulus to other cardiac cells. This characteristic is shared by all cardiac cells, because these cells are connected together to form a syncytium (they function collectively as a unit).

Contractility is also referred to as *rhythmicity* and is the ability of cardiac cells to shorten and cause cardiac muscle contraction in response to an electrical stimulus. Contractility can be thought of as the coordination of contractions of cardiac muscle cells to produce a regular heartbeat. Cardiac contractility can be strengthened through the administration of certain medications, such as dopamine and epinephrine.

MAJOR ELECTROLYTES THAT AFFECT CARDIAC FUNCTION

Because myocardial cells are bathed in electrolyte solutions, both mechanical and electrical cardiac function is influenced by electrolyte imbalances. An electrolyte is a substance or compound whose molecules dissociate into charged components, or ions, when placed in water, producing positively and negatively charged ions. An ion with a positive charge is called a *cation* and an ion with a negative charge is called an *anion*.

The three major cations that affect cardiac function are potassium (K), sodium (Na), and calcium (Ca). Magnesium (Mg) is also an important cation. Potassium, magnesium, and calcium are intracellular (inside the cell) cations, while sodium is an extracellular (outside the cell) cation.

Potassium performs a major function in cardiac depolarization and repolarization. An increase in potassium blood levels is known as *hyperkalemia*, while a potassium deficit is termed *hypokalemia*. Sodium plays a vital part in depolarization of the myocardium. An increase in sodium blood levels is known as *hypernatremia,* while a sodium deficit is termed *hyponatremia.* Calcium renders an important function in myocardial depolarization and myocardial contraction. An increase in calcium blood levels is known as *hypercalcemia,* while a calcium deficit is called *hypocalcemia.*

MOVEMENT OF IONS

Let's think now about the cardiac cell at rest or in its resting state. Normally there exists an ionic difference on the two sides of the cell membrane. In this state, potassium ion concentration is greater inside the cell than outside and sodium ion concentration is greater outside the cell than inside. Potassium ions can diffuse through the membrane more readily than can sodium ions. By means of an active (or energized) mechanism of transport called the **sodium-potassium exchange pump,** potassium and sodium ions are moved in and out of the cell through the cell membrane. During the polarized or resting state, the inside of the cell is electrically negative relative to the outside of the cell. For purposes of discussions in the upcoming chapters of this text, it should be noted that, during this resting period, a baseline or isoelectric line is recorded on the EKG strip.

CARDIAC DEPOLARIZATION

When an impulse develops and spreads throughout the myocardium, certain changes occur in the heart muscle fibers. These changes are referred to as *cardiac depolarization* and *cardiac repolarization.* In order to accurately and reasonably understand EKG interpretation, one must understand the concept of cardiac depolarization and repolarization.

First, let's define a few terms that will be utilized in this discussion.

Resting membrane potential   the state of a cardiac cell in which the inside of the cell membrane is negative when compared to the outside of the cell membrane; exists when cardiac cells are in the resting state.

Action potential   a change in polarity; a five-phase cycle that produces changes in the cell membrane's electrical charge; caused by stimulation of myocardial cells that extends across the myocardium; propagated in an all-or-none fashion.

Syncytium   cardiac muscle cell groups that are connected together and function collectively as a unit.

Polarized state   the resting state of a cardiac cell, wherein the inside of the cell is electrically negative relative to the outside of the cell.

Depolarization   an electrical occurrence normally expected to result in myocardial contraction; involves the movement of ions across cardiac cell membranes, resulting in positive polarity inside the cell membrane.

Repolarization   process whereby the depolarized cell is polarized and positive charges are again on the outside and negative charges on the inside of the cell; a return to the resting state.

For the sake of clarity, cardiac depolarization may be thought of as the period during which sodium ions rush into the cell, changing the interior charge to positive, after a myocardial cell has been stimulated. Recall now that this change of polarity is referred to as the *action potential*. In an effort to change the interior cell polarity to positive, calcium also slowly enters into the cell. This activated state of the myocardial cells now spreads through the syncytium, followed closely by myocardial muscle contraction. This difference in the electric charge or polarity on the outside of the cell membrane results in the flow of electric current, which is recorded as waveforms on the EKG (see Fig. 3-1).

CARDIAC REPOLARIZATION

At the end of cardiac depolarization, sodium actively returns to the outside of the cell and potassium returns to the inside of the cell. This exchange takes place via the sodium-potassium exchange pump. The cell has now returned to the recovered or repolarized state. The cardiac cell is now ready to be stimulated again. Repolarization is a slower process than depolarization.

It may be helpful to recall that the polarized cell is in the resting state, the depolarization of the cell is utilizing its action potential, and the repo-

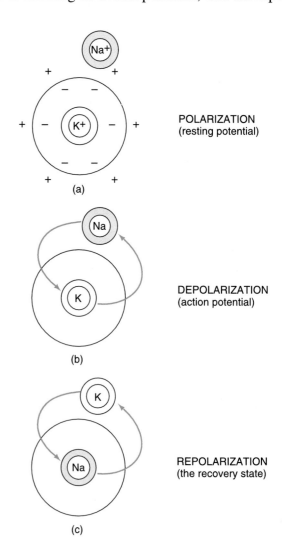

Figure 3-1 Ion shifts during depolarization and repolarization.

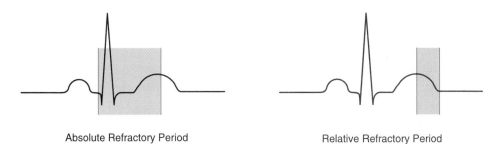

Absolute Refractory Period   Relative Refractory Period

Figure 3-2 Refractory periods.

larized cell is in the recovery phase. It should be noted that the last area to be depolarized is the first area to be repolarized in normal, healthy cardiac muscle.

REFRACTORY PERIODS

Like all other excitable tissue, cardiac muscle tissue has a refractory period that attempts to ensure that the muscle is totally relaxed before another action potential or depolarization can be initiated. The refractory period of atrial muscle is much shorter (approximately 0.15 sec) than that of ventricular muscle (approximately 0.25 to 0.3 sec). Thus the rate of atrial contractions can potentially be much faster than that of the ventricles.

After electrical impulse stimulation and myocardial contraction, the cardiac cells enjoy a brief resting period. As we learned earlier in this discussion, this period of rest is referred to as *cardiac repolarization*. During this state of repolarization, the heart goes through two stages: the absolute refractory period and the relative refractory period (see Fig. 3-2). During the majority of the process of repolarization, the cardiac cell is unable to respond to a new electrical stimulus. In addition, the cardiac cell cannot spontaneously depolarize. This stage of the cell is referred to as the *absolute refractory period*. Remember that, regardless of the strength of the stimulus, the cardiac cell cannot be stimulated to depolarize during this time. The absolute refractory period corresponds with the beginning of the QRS complex to the peak of the T wave on the EKG strip.

The second part of the refractory period follows the absolute refractory period and is referred to as the *relative refractory period*. The relative refractory period is the period when repolarization is almost complete and the cardiac cell can be stimulated to contract prematurely if the stimulus is much stronger than normal. On the EKG strip, the relative refractory period corresponds with the downslope of the T wave. The relative refractory period is also known as the *vulnerable period* of the cardiac cells during repolarization.

REVIEW QUESTIONS: CHAPTER 3

1. The primary functions of the myocardial working cells include:

   a. Automaticity

   b. Regeneration

    c. Contraction and relaxation

    d. Impulse propagation

2. The ability of cardiac pacemaker cells to spontaneously generate their own electrical impulses without external (or nervous) stimulation is known as:

    a. Automaticity

    b. Contractility

    c. Conductility

    d. Action potential

3. This characteristic is specific to the pacemaker cells sites of the electrical conduction system (i.e., the SA node, the AV junction, and the Purkinje network fibers):

    a. Automaticity

    b. Contractility

    c. Conductility

    d. Excitability

4. The ability of cardiac cells to respond to an electrical stimulus is referred to as:

    a. Automaticity

    b. Contractility

    c. Conductility

    d. Excitability

5. Excitability is also referred to as:

    a. Irritability

    b. Automaticity

    c. Contractility

    d. Conductility

6. The ability of cardiac cells to receive an electrical stimulus and then to transmit the stimulus to other cardiac cells is known as:

    a. Irritability

    b. Automaticity

    c. Contractility

    d. Conductivity

7. Conductivity is a characteristic shared by all cardiac cells.

    a. True

    b. False

8. Cardiac muscle cell groups that function collectively as a unit are known as:

    a. Syncytia

b. Refractory

c. Electrical

d. Bundles

9. Repolarization is a slower process than depolarization.

a. True

b. False

10. The period when repolarization is almost complete and the cardiac cell can be stimulated to contract prematurely if the stimulus is stronger than normal is known as the:

a. Relative refractory period

b. Absolute refractory period

c. Action potential phase

d. Active depolarization

4

THE ELECTRICAL
CONDUCTION SYSTEM

Objectives

Upon completion of this chapter, the student will be able to:

1. Identify the location of the following:
   a. SA node
   b. Internodal pathways
   c. AV node
   d. Bundle of His
   e. AV junction
   f. Bundle branches
   g. Purkinje network
2. Describe the function of the following:
   a. SA node

   b. Internodal pathways
   c. AV node
   d. Bundle of His
   e. AV junction
   f. Bundle branches
   g. Purkinje network
3. Relate the normal path of an impulse traveling through the electrical conduction system

The heart's pacing (or conducting) system (see Fig. 4-1) is responsible for the electrical activity that controls each normal heartbeat. This unique system consists of specialized cells and fibers that are collectively known as **nodes** or **bundles.** These nodes and bundles are relatively small and are located primarily beneath the **endocardium** (the innermost lining of the chambers of the heart). Specialized parts of this system are capable of initiating electrical activity automatically and can act as pacemakers for the heart.

A thorough understanding of the electrical conduction system of the heart is an essential component of learning and understanding an EKG strip. While it is important to note that the 3-lead EKG strip is representative of **only** the electrical activity of the heart, the student must also understand that the clinician cannot determine the mechanical activity of the patient's heart by merely

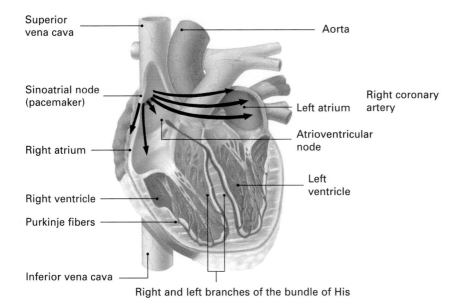

Superior vena cava

Aorta

Sinoatrial node (pacemaker)

Right coronary artery

Left atrium

Right atrium

Atrioventricular node

Left ventricle

Right ventricle

Purkinje fibers

Inferior vena cava

Right and left branches of the bundle of His

Figure 4-1 The cardiac conduction system.

looking at a 3-lead EKG strip. However, by incorporating the basic knowledge of 12-lead EKG interpretation, you will gain more knowledge about the changes occurring in the myocardium when a patient is experiencing a myocardial infarction, specifically regarding the area of myocardial tissue involvement as well as which coronary artery is most likely involved.

In order to begin to determine that an EKG strip is abnormal, the student must first understand the normal parameters for the graphic representation of the electrical activity of the heart. It is to that end that this chapter is presented. In this chapter, you will recall the locations of the pacemakers and conducting fibers, as well as how they function during a normal heartbeat. Table 4-1 gives an overview of the electrical conduction system of the heart.

SA Node

The sinoatrial (SA) node is located in the upper posterior portion of the right atrial wall of the heart, near the opening of the superior vena cava. The node is made up of a cluster of hundreds of cells that comprise a knot of modified heart muscle that is capable of generating impulses that travel throughout the muscle fibers of both atria, resulting in depolarization.

TABLE 4-1 REVIEW OF THE ELECTRICAL CONDUCTION SYSTEM OF THE HEART				
SA Node	Internodal Pathways	AV Junction (AV Node and Bundle)	Bundle Branches	Purkinje Network
Firing rate of 60–100 BPM	Transfer impulse from the SA node throughout the atria to the AV junction	Slows impulse; intrinsic firing rate of 40–60 BPM	Two main branches (left and right); transmit impulse to ventricles	Spreads impulse throughout the ventricles; intrinsic firing rate of 20–40 BPM

The SA node is commonly referred to as the primary pacemaker of the heart because it normally depolarizes more rapidly than any other part of the conduction system. The normal range or firing rate of the heart's primary pacemaker (SA node) is 60 to 100 beats per minute (BPM).

If, for a variety of reasons, the dominant pacemaker fails to fire within the normal range, another group of specialized tissues, such as the atrioventricular tissue or the Purkinje network of fibers, will assume the duties of the pacemaker. These backup pacemakers are arranged in a waterfall fashion. Depolarization and resultant myocardial contraction occurs as the impulse leaves the SA node and travels further down the path of the electrical conduction system.

INTERNODAL PATHWAYS

Three internodal tracts or pathways receive the electrical impulse as it exits the SA node. These tracts distribute the electrical impulse throughout the atria and transmit the impulse from the SA node to the atrioventricular (AV) node. The internodal tracts consist of anterior, middle, and posterior divisions. A group of interatrial fibers contained in the left atrium is referred to as *Bachmann's bundle*. Bachmann's bundle is a subdivision of the anterior internodal tract. This specialized group of cardiac fibers conducts electrical activity from the SA node to the left atrium.

AV NODE

The AV node is located on the floor of the right atrium just above the tricuspid valve. At the level of the AV node, the electrical activity is delayed by approximately 0.05 second. This delay allows for atrial contraction and a more complete filling of the ventricles. The AV node includes three regions: the AV junctional tissue between the atria and node, the nodal area, and the AV junctional tissue between the node and the bundle of His. In the normal heart, the AV node is the only pathway for conduction of atrial electrical impulses to the ventricles.

AV JUNCTION

The region where the internodal pathways leading from the SA node join the bundle of His is called the *AV junction*. Similar to the SA node, the AV junctional tissue contains fibers that can depolarize spontaneously, forming an electrical impulse that can spread to the heart chambers. Therefore, if the SA node fails or slows below its normal range, the AV junctional tissues can initiate electrical activity and thus assume the role of a secondary pacemaker.

BUNDLE OF HIS

The conduction pathway that leads out of the AV node was described by a German physician, Wilhelm His, in 1893 and has subsequently been referred to as the *bundle of His*. The bundle of His is approximately 15 millimeters long and lies at the top of the interventricular septum. The interventricular septum is the wall between the right and left ventricles.

The bundle of His is also traditionally referred to as the *common bundle*. This bundle of specialized cells contains pacemaker cells that have the ability to self-initiate electrical activity at an intrinsic firing rate of 40 to 60 beats per minute.

BUNDLE BRANCHES

The bundle of His divides into two main branches at the top of the interventricular septum. These branches are the right bundle branch and the left bundle branch. The primary function of the bundle branches is to conduct electrical activity from the bundle of His down to the Purkinje network. A long, thin structure lying beneath the endocardium, the right bundle branch runs down the right side of the interventricular septum and terminates at the papillary muscles in the right ventricle. This bundle branch functions to carry electrical impulses to the right ventricle. Shorter than the right bundle branch, the left bundle branch divides into pathways that spread from the left side of the interventricular septum and throughout the left ventricle. The two main divisions of the left bundle branch are called **fascicles.** The anterior fascicle carries electrical impulses to the anterior wall of the left ventricle; the posterior fascicle spreads the impulses to the posterior ventricular wall. The bundle branches continue to divide until they finally terminate in the Purkinje fibers.

PURKINJE NETWORK

Bundle branches lead to a network of small conduction fibers that spread throughout the ventricles. These fibers were first described in 1787 by Johannes E. Purkinje, a Czechoslovakian physiologist. This network of fibers carries electrical impulses directly to ventricular muscle cells. The fibers that connect with the Purkinje fibers start in the atrioventricular node in the right atrium of the heart.

Purkinje fibers can only be identified with the aid of a microscope, but are larger in diameter than ordinary cardiac muscle fibers. Ventricular contraction is facilitated by the rapid spread of the electrical impulse through the left and right bundle branches and Purkinje fibers into the ventricular muscle. Purkinje network fibers possess the intrinsic ability to serve as pacemakers. The firing rate of the Purkinje pacemaker fibers is normally within the range of 20 to 40 beats per minute.

REVIEW QUESTIONS: CHAPTER 4

1. The SA node is located in the:
   a. Right atrium
   b. Right ventricle

    c. Purkinje fiber tract

    d. Atrioventricular septum

2. The AV node is located in the:

    a. Right atrium

    b. Left ventricle

    c. Purkinje fiber tract

    d. Atrioventricular septum

3. The intrinsic firing rate of the AV junction is:

    a. 15–25 BPM

    b. 25–35 BPM

    c. 35–45 BPM

    d. 40–60 BPM

4. The intrinsic rate of the SA node in the adult is:

    a. 20–60 BPM

    b. 40–80 BPM

    c. 60–100 BPM

    d. 80–100 BPM

5. The electrocardiogram is used to:

    a. Determine pulse rate

    b. Detect valvular dysfunction

    c. Evaluate electrical activity in the heart

    d. Determine whether the heart is beating

6. The normal conduction pattern of the heart follows:

    1. SA node

    2. Purkinje fibers

    3. Bundle of His

    4. AV node

    5. Bundle branches

    6. Internodal pathways

    a. 1, 2, 3, 5, 6, 4

    b. 1, 6, 4, 3, 5, 2

    c. 1, 6, 4, 2, 3, 5

    d. 6, 1, 5, 4, 6, 2

7. The primary pacemaker of the heart is the:

    a. AV node

    b. SA node

    c. Purkinje fibers

    d. SV node

8. The bundle of His is also traditionally referred to as the:

   a. Lesser bundle

   b. Chordae tendineae

   c. Common bundle

   d. Coronary sinus

9. The fibers of the Purkinje network can only be identified with the aid of a microscope.

   a. True

   b. False

10. The region where the internodal pathways leading from the SA node join the bundle of His is called the:

   a. Bachmann's bundle

   b. AV junction

   c. SA junction

   d. Common bundle

5

THE ELECTROCARDIOGRAM

Objectives

Upon completion of this chapter, the student will be able to:

1. Describe the types of EKG leads
2. Identify and explain the grids and markings on a representative strip of EKG graph paper
3. Discuss the electrical basis of the electrocardiogram
4. Describe the relationship of the following EKG waveforms to the electrical events in the heart:

   a. P wave
   b. PR Interval
   c. QRS complex
   d. J point
   e. ST segment
   f. T wave

The medical use of the electrocardiogram dates back less than a century, to around the year 1900. Modern technology has brought us very far in the past 100 years, to the point where almost every emergency department and prehospital advanced life support unit has equipment suitable for obtaining either a 3-lead or a 12-lead EKG on a patient whenever and wherever indicated. The most significant lesson that you will learn while traveling through this textbook centers not on the EKG tracing, but on the clinical picture of your patient. You must continually ask yourself, "How is this rhythm clinically significant to the patient?" Regardless of the pattern observed on the oscilloscope or EKG static strip, your patient's condition is and must be your primary concern. Keep this important fact in mind, and your patient's best interests will always be served.

ELECTRICAL BASIS OF THE EKG

In Chapter 4 we explored the components and functions of the heart's electrical conduction system. Based on that knowledge, we should understand that the heart generates electrical activity in the body; thus the body can be thought of as a major conductor of electrical activity. This electrical activity can be sensed by electrodes placed on the skin's surface and can be recorded in the form of an electrocardiogram. Cardiac monitors depict the heart's electrical impulses as patterns of waves on the monitor screen or oscilloscope. Because electrical impulses present on the skin surface are very low in voltage, the impulses must be amplified by the EKG machine. The printed record of the electrical activity of the heart is called a *rhythm strip* or an *EKG strip* (see Fig. 5-1).

EKG LEADS

As we discussed earlier in this chapter, the cardiac monitor receives electrical impulses from the patient's heart through electrodes placed on particular areas of the body. An electrode is an adhesive pad that contains conductive gel and is designed to be attached to the patient's skin. These electrodes are then connected to the monitor or EKG machine by wires called *leads*. These wires are generally color coded in order to be user-friendly.

In EKG monitoring, the term *lead* is sometimes used in two different contexts. Another meaning of this term is referenced when speaking of a

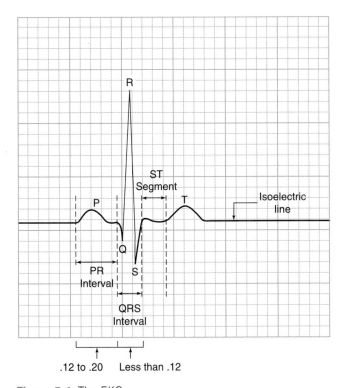

Figure 5-1 The EKG.

pair of electrodes, such as chest Lead I, II, modified chest lead, and so on. In the latter usage, the term is generally capitalized.

In order for the monitor or EKG machine to receive a clear picture of the electrical impulses generated by the heart's electrical conduction system, there must be a positive, a negative, and a ground lead. You should remember that the electrical current of the heart flows from right to left. The ground lead serves to minimize outside electrical interference.

The exact portion of the heart being visualized depends in large part on the placement of the electrodes. It may be helpful to envision the heart as an object placed on a pedestal around which a person can move while taking photographs (different views) from all angles. This analogy would describe the 12-lead EKG, whereas only one snapshot or view of the heart would represent the 3-lead EKG.

The 12-lead EKG is commonly used in hospitals and clinics, while the 3-lead EKG is typically used in the field. In some areas of the country, 12-lead EKGs are being utilized regularly in the prehospital setting to aid in screening patients who are potential candidates for thrombolytic therapy. It is important to note that the 3-lead EKG is sufficient for detecting life-threatening dysrhythmias.

Lead II and the modified chest lead (MCL) are the most common leads used for cardiac monitoring because of their ability to visualize P waves. Leads I, II and III are known as *bipolar leads,* which means that these leads have one positive electrode and one negative electrode. Bipolar leads are sometimes referred to as *limb leads.* Table 5-1 details the placement of electrodes of the three bipolar leads on certain areas of the body.

An imaginary inverted triangle is formed around the heart by proper placement of the bipolar leads. This triangle is referred to as *Einthoven's triangle* (see Fig. 5-2). The top of the triangle is formed by Lead I, the right side of the triangle is formed by Lead II, and the left side of the triangle is formed by Lead III. Each lead represents a different look at, or view of, the heart.

You may recall the discussion of topographic anatomy in your basic anatomy courses, and you may remember that a *plane* refers to an imaginary surface. You should be aware that the 12-lead EKG views the heart in two distinct planes. These planes include the horizontal and frontal planes (see Fig. 5-3). The vector (V) leads look at the horizontal plane and the limb leads look at the frontal plane.

TABLE 5-1 BIPOLAR LEAD PLACEMENT		
Lead	Positive Electrode	Negative Electrode
I	Left arm	Right arm
II	Left leg	Right arm
III	Left leg	Left arm

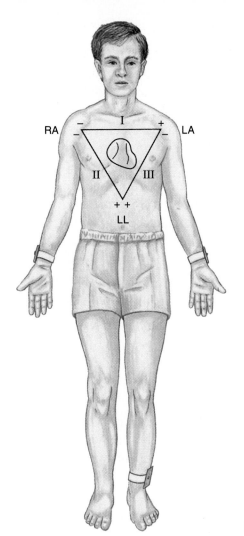

Figure 5-2 Einthoven's triangle.

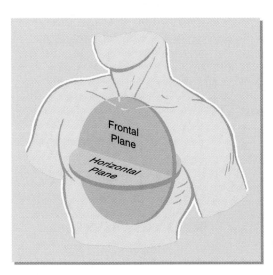

Figure 5-3 Planes: frontal and horizontal.

Standard Limb Leads

Leads I, II, and III are the first leads of a 12-lead EKG (standard limb leads). At this point, it is important to emphasize the significance of the specific placement of leads (see Fig. 5-4). The left arm lead should be placed at a location between the left shoulder and wrist, being sure to stay away from bony prominences, as bone is a poor conductor of electricity. The right lead should be placed between the right shoulder and wrist. The left leg lead should be placed between the left hip and ankle, away from bony prominences. The right leg lead is placed between the right hip and ankle and is sometimes utilized as an additional ground lead.

If you feel obligated or if local protocol dictates that you place the limb leads on the trunk, rather than the extremities, you should note this action on the 12-lead strip, as further evaluation may be affected by this decision. In other words, if placement of the limb leads deviates from the normal position (extremities), then this positioning may effect the direction of the axis. Axis deviation will be discussed in detail in Chapter 14.

Augmented Limb Leads

In order to simplify the explanation of the augmented limb leads (see Table 5-2), we suggest that you begin by viewing the heart as the focal point of this discussion. In the first three leads (standard), the negative-to-positive current flows from the limbs through the heart. However, in the augmented

Limb Lead Placement

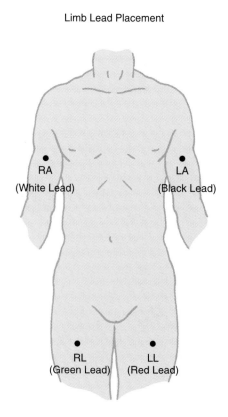

Figure 5-4 Standard limb leads.

TABLE 5-2 AUGMENTED LEADS

Augmented Leads	Position of Flow
aVR—augmented voltage, right arm	From the heart to the right arm
aVL—augmented voltage, left arm	From the heart to the left arm
aVF—augmented voltage, left foot	From the heart to the left foot

leads, the current flows from the heart outward to the extremities; hence the name *augmented* or *extended from the heart*. Augmented leads are also referred to as *unipolar* (having only one true pole) leads. It may also be valuable for you to understand that the EKG machine must boost (or raise) amplification due to the positions of these leads.

Chest Leads

The chest leads are also unipolar and comprise the last six leads on the 12-lead EKG (see Fig. 5-5). These leads look at the heart via the horizontal (or transverse) plane. These leads are also called *precordial* or vector (V) leads. Proper placement of the V leads (see Table 5-3) is critically important to the correct interpretation of the 12-lead EKG strip. Specific guidelines should be established and followed each time a 12-lead EKG is obtained— merely guessing about placement is not allowed!!

You should become proficient in correct lead placement in order to assure that 12-lead EKG interpretation is consistent for all patients. It is important that the patient's skin be properly prepared before attaching the leads. You should complete the following steps:

1. Clean the area with an alcohol swab and allow the area to dry.

2. Shave excess hair as indicated.

3. If the patient is diaphoretic, attempt to dry the area or use spray antiperspirant on the area to effect drying.

4. Make sure the leads are properly placed, including measuring each lead. This is imperative! Improper lead placement can affect R wave progression through the V leads. (R wave progression is discussed later in this chapter.)

5. Make sure that the conductive gel is pliable in order to ensure proper conduction.

You should realize that, although we refer to the "12-lead EKG," only 10 cardiac monitor leads are required (4 limb leads and 6 chest leads) to obtain the tracing. (See Fig. 5-6 for a sample tracing.) Only by completing each of the steps just discussed in an efficient and timely manner can you ensure that each 12-lead EKG strip is done consistently.

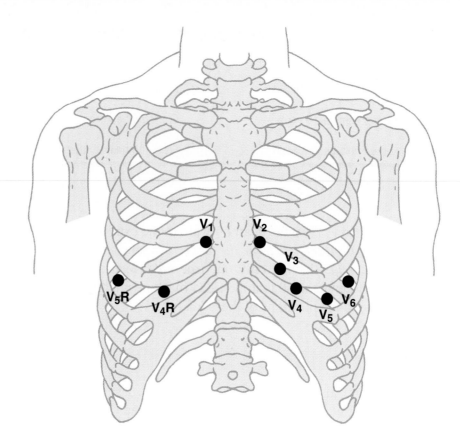

V$_1$—4th intercostal space, right of the sternum
V$_2$—4th intercostal space, left of the sternum
V$_3$—5th intercostal space, halfway between V$_2$ and V$_4$
V$_4$—5th intercostal space, left midclavicular line
V$_5$—5th intercostal space, left anterior axillary line
V$_6$—5th intercostal space, left midaxillary line
V$_4$R—5th intercostal space, right midclavicular line
V$_5$R—5th intercostal space, right anterior axillary line

Figure 5-5 Chest lead placement.

TABLE 5-3 CHEST LEAD PLACEMENT	
Lead	Placement
V$_1$	Fourth intercostal space, just to the right of the sternum
V$_2$	Fourth intercostal space, just to the left of the sternum
V$_3$	Between V$_2$ and V$_4$
V$_4$	Fifth intercostal space, midclavicular line
V$_5$	Anterior axillary line, level with V$_4$
V$_6$	Midaxillary line, level with V$_4$ and V$_5$

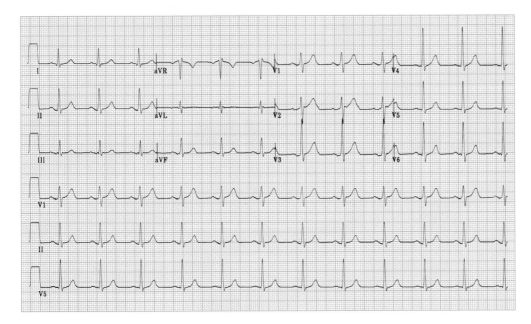

Figure 5-6 12-lead EKG.

EKG Graph Paper

Electrocardiographic paper is arranged as a series of horizontal and vertical lines printed on graph paper and provides a printed record of cardiac electrical activity. This paper is standardized to allow for consistency in EKG rhythm strip analysis. EKG paper leaves the machine at a constant speed of 25 millimeters per second for a standard 12-lead EKG.

Both time and amplitude (or voltage) are measured on the graph paper. Time is measured on the horizontal line, while amplitude or voltage is measured on the vertical line. The vertical axis reflects millivolts (two large squares = 1 mV; 1 mV = 10 mm). The millivolt is the standard calibration for 12-lead EKGs. EKG graph paper is divided into small squares, each of which is 1 millimeter in height and width and represents a time interval of 0.04 second. Darker lines further divide the paper every fifth square, both vertically and horizontally. Each of these large squares measures 5 millimeters in height and 5 millimeters in width and represents a time interval of 0.20 second. There are five small squares in each large square; therefore 5 (small squares) × 0.04 second = 0.20 second. The squares on the EKG paper represent the measurement of the length of time required for the electrical impulse to traverse a specific part of the heart (see Fig. 5-7). Proper interpretation of EKG rhythms is dependent in part on understanding the time increments as represented on EKG paper.

EKG Waveforms

A *wave* or *waveform* recorded on an EKG strip refers to movement away from the baseline, or isoelectric line, and is represented as a positive deflection (above the isoelectric line) or a negative deflection (below the isoelectric line). The baseline is the straight line seen on an EKG strip and represents the beginning and ending point of all waves.

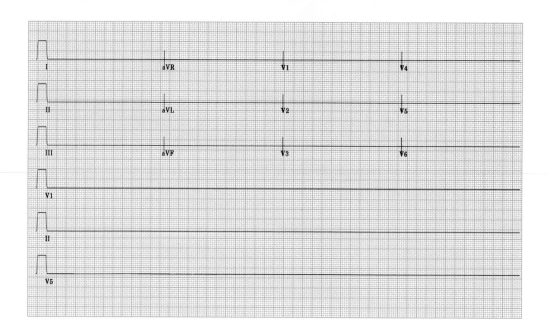

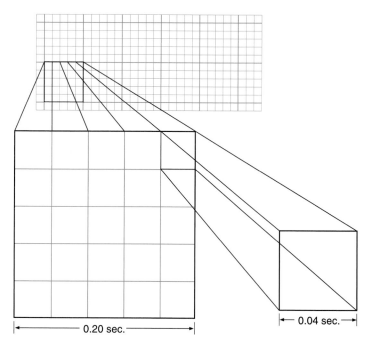

Figure 5-7 EKG paper and its markings.

As the electrical impulse leaves the sinoatrial (SA) node, waveforms are produced on the graph paper. One complete cardiac cycle is represented on graph paper by five major waves: the P wave, the Q, R, and S waves (normally referred to as the *QRS complex*), and the T wave.

P Wave

As we discussed in Chapter 4, the SA node fires first during a normal cardiac cycle. This firing event sends the electrical impulse outward to stimulate both atria and manifests as the P wave (see Fig. 5-8). When observed on a Lead II EKG strip, the P wave is a smooth, rounded upward deflection.

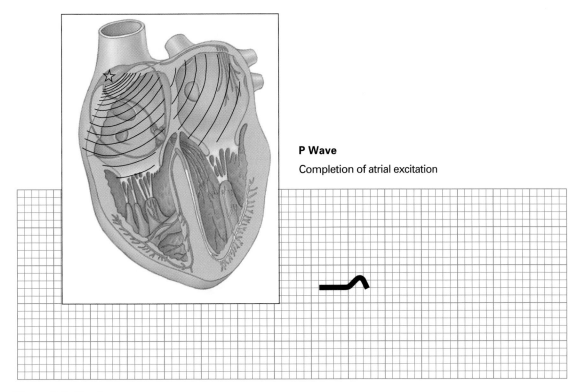

P Wave

Completion of atrial excitation

Figure 5-8 The P wave.

The P wave represents depolarization of both the left and right atria and is approximately 0.10 second in length.

PR Interval

Sometimes abbreviated as **PRI,** the PR Interval represents the time interval necessary for the impulse to travel from the SA node through the internodal pathways in the atria and downward to the ventricles. In simpler terms, the PRI is said to be representative of the distance from the beginning of the P wave to the beginning of the QRS complex. The normal PR Interval is measured as three to five small squares on the EKG graph paper and is 0.12 to 0.20 second in length (see Fig. 5-9).

QRS Complex

The QRS complex (see Fig. 5-10) consists of the Q, R, and S waves and represents the conduction of the electrical impulse from the bundle of His throughout the ventricular muscle, or ventricular depolarization. The Q wave is seen as the first downward deflection following the PRI. The R wave is the first upward deflection of the QRS complex and is normally the largest deflection seen in chest Leads I and II. Immediately following the R wave is a downward deflection, which is called the S wave.

The QRS complex is measured from the beginning of the Q wave to the point where the S wave meets the baseline. Normally, the QRS complex measures less than 0.12 second, or less than three small squares on the EKG

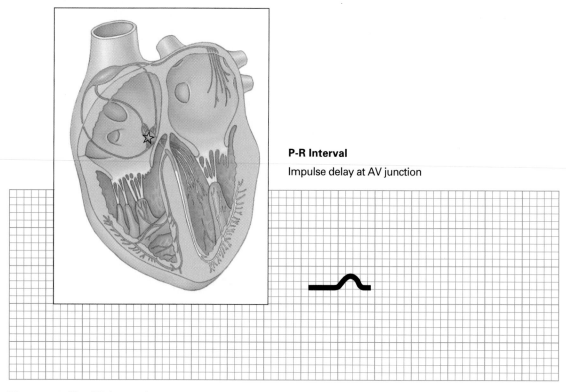

P-R Interval

Impulse delay at AV junction

Figure 5-9 The PR Interval.

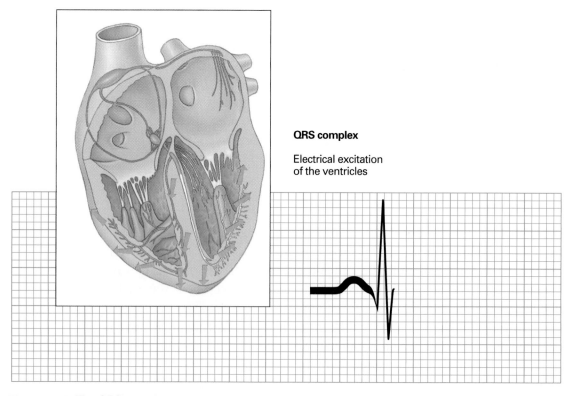

QRS complex

Electrical excitation
of the ventricles

Figure 5-10 The QRS complex.

graph paper. It should be noted that the shape of the QRS complex varies from individual to individual and that all three waves are not always present.

J Point

The point at which the QRS complex meets the ST segment is known as the J point (see Fig. 5-11) and is an important landmark in 12-lead EKG interpretation. Generally, an elevation or depression of 1 millimeter or more (above or below the isoelectric line) may be indicative of myocardial injury or ischemia. Consideration of ST segment elevation or depression begins with the analysis of the J point.

ST Segment

The time interval during which the ventricles are depolarized and ventricular repolarization begins is called the ST segment. Normally the ST segment is isoelectric, or consistent with the baseline. In certain cardiac disease processes, the ST segment may be elevated or depressed due to ischemia and/or infarction. Elevation of the ST segment is one of the major EKG changes appreciated in acute myocardial infarction.

T Wave

Following the ST segment is the T wave (see Fig. 5-12), which represents ventricular repolarization. The T wave is normally seen as a slightly asymmetrical, slightly rounded, positive deflection. Recall now that ventricular repolarization is an electrical event with no associated activity of the ventricular musculature. The T wave is often referred to as the *resting phase* of the cardiac cycle.

Recall also that the refractory periods, both absolute and relative, are in place during the EKG representation of the T wave and thus the heart may be vulnerable to strong impulses that may lead to ventricular dysrhythmias. The T wave may be either elevated or depressed in the presence of current or previous cardiac ischemia. Normally one complete cardiac cycle is represented by the PQRST pattern (see Table 5-4).

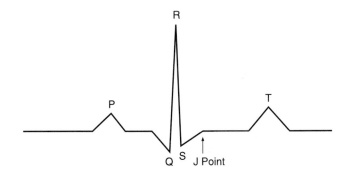

Figure 5-11 The J point.

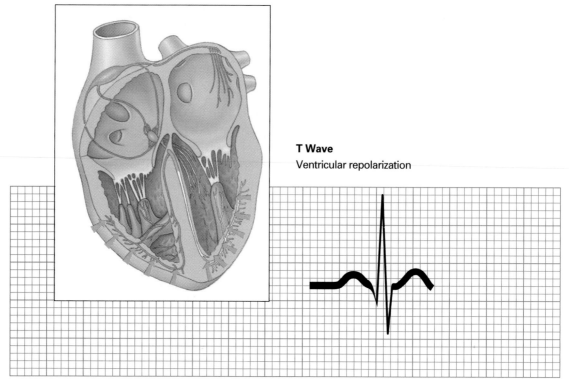

T Wave
Ventricular repolarization

Figure 5-12 The T wave.

STANDARD 12-LEAD EKG WAVEFORMS

The understanding of normal 12-lead EKG waveform configurations is imperative in the correct interpretation of the 12-lead EKG (see Fig. 5-13). Specifically, you should remember that in limb Leads I, II, and III all waveforms should be positively deflected (upright). In the augmented leads (aVR, aVL, aVF) the deflection of waveforms varies. In the aVR lead, all waveforms are negatively deflected; however in aVL, the P wave and T wave are negatively deflected, but the QRS complex is biphasic (waveforms are equally positive and negative in deflection). In aVF, all waveforms are positively deflected. In the precordial or chest leads, all P and T waves are positively deflected; however, the QRS waveform initiates as a negative deflection and progresses until it becomes absolutely positive in lead V_6.

If you study Table 5-5, you will note that the R wave of the QRS complex initially appears as a negative deflection in V_1 and progresses through the V leads to become a totally positive deflection in V_6. This concept is known as normal **R wave progression.**

TABLE 5-4 SUMMARY OF EKG WAVEFORMS AND CORRELATING CARDIAC EVENTS	
P wave represents	Atrial depolarization
QRS complex represents	Ventricular depolarization; atrial repolarization (hidden in QRS complex)
T wave represents	Ventricular repolarization

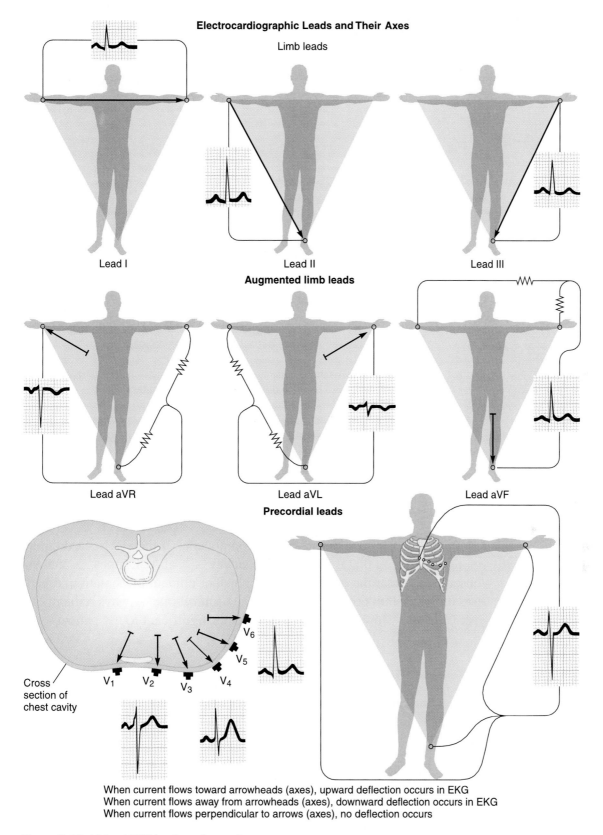

Figure 5-13 12-lead EKG leads and waveforms.

When current flows toward arrowheads (axes), upward deflection occurs in EKG
When current flows away from arrowheads (axes), downward deflection occurs in EKG
When current flows perpendicular to arrows (axes), no deflection occurs

TABLE 5-5 NORMAL 12-LEAD EKG WAVEFORMS	
Lead I	P, Q, R, S, and T waveforms are positively deflected (upright)
Lead II	P, Q, R, S, and T waveforms are positively deflected (upright)
Lead III	P, Q, R, S, and T waveforms are positively deflected (upright)
aVR	P, Q, R, S, and T waveforms are negatively deflected
aVL	P and T waves are negative; QRS waveform is biphasic
aVF	P, Q, R, S, and T waveforms are positively deflected (upright)
V_1	P and T waves are positively deflected; QRS waveform initiates as a negative deflection
V_2	P and T waves are positively deflected; QRS waveform is primarily a negative deflection with minimal positive deflection
V_3	P and T waves are positively deflected; QRS waveform is primarily biphasic with negative deflection being predominant
V_4	P and T waves are positively deflected; QRS waveform is primarily biphasic with positive deflection being predominant
V_5	P and T waves are positively deflected; QRS waveform is primarily positive with slight negative deflection
V_6	P and T waves are positively deflected; QRS waveform is positively deflected

Now that we have discussed the components of the electrocardiogram, let us remind you that it is imperative, always . . . at ALL times . . . that you observe and treat the patient based on his/her clinical presentation, regardless of the rhythm being observed on the oscilloscope! Always remember to ask yourself, "How is this rhythm clinically significant to my patient?"

REVIEW QUESTIONS: CHAPTER 5

1. Ventricular diastole refers to ventricular:
   a. Contraction
   b. Relaxation
   c. Filling time
   d. Pressure ratio

2. The single-lead electrocardiogram is used primarily to:
   a. Determine cardiac output
   b. Detect valvular dysfunction
   c. Evaluate electrical activity in the heart
   d. Detect left-to-right conduction disorders

3. The PR interval should normally be _____ or smaller.
   a. 0.10 sec
   b. 0.12 sec
   c. 0.08 sec
   d. 0.20 sec

4. The QRS interval should normally be _____ or smaller.
   a. 0.20 sec
   b. 0.12 sec
   c. 0.18 sec
   d. 0.36 sec

5. The QRS complex is produced when the:
   a. Ventricles repolarize
   b. Ventricles depolarize
   c. Ventricles contract
   d. Both b and c

6. The normal conduction pattern of the heart follows:
   1. SA node
   2. Purkinje fibers
   3. Bundle of His
   4. AV node
   5. Bundle branches
   6. Internodal pathways

   a. 1, 5, 2, 4, 6, 3
   b. 1, 6, 4, 3, 5, 2
   c. 1, 4, 3, 6, 5, 2
   d. 1, 2, 3, 4, 5, 6

7. The T wave on the EKG strip represents:
   a. Rest period
   b. Bundle of His
   c. Atrial contraction
   d. Ventricular contraction

8. The point at which the QRS complex meets the ST segment is known as the:
   a. Delta wave
   b. End point
   c. J point
   d. Vector

9. When interpreting dysrhythmias, the health care provider should remember that the most important key is the:

   a. PR Interval

   b. Rate and rhythm

   c. Presence of dysrhythmias

   d. Patient's clinical appearance

10. How many cardiac monitor pads are utilized when obtaining a 12-lead EKG?

    a. 10

    b. 12

    c. 3

    d. 6

6

INTERPRETATION OF EKG STRIPS

Objectives

Upon completion of this chapter, the student will be able to:

1. Describe a basic approach for interpretation of EKG strips
2. Explain the five steps used in interpretation of EKG strips
3. Explain how to calculate heart rate, given a 6-second strip
4. Explain the 5 + 3 approach, including:
   a. ST elevation
   b. ST depression
   c. Q wave

This is a very significant chapter for you to master in order to fully understand EKG interpretation. The preceding chapters in this text are essential building blocks leading up to this chapter. The upcoming chapters will focus on application of the rules mastered in this chapter. Therefore, this chapter is critical to your understanding of proper interpretation of EKG rhythm strips.

For many years now, we have explained to students that the key to learning, interpreting, and, most importantly, understanding dysrhythmias is a systematic approach that must be used each and every time a strip is analyzed. Frankly speaking, we do not really expect you to believe that all health care professionals who have been practicing their craft for many years now **always** apply this five-step, systematic approach for every strip they see. However, you are utilizing this book because you wish to learn how to effortlessly interpret dysrhythmias using both 3-lead and 12-lead strips. Keep in mind that, while you are learning this skill, memorization will not suffice. You must learn and apply this systematic approach to EKG analysis. When you look at a strip, think about and apply these five steps and you should be successful in mastering the art of EKG analysis.

GENERAL RULES

Here are a few basic rules that will assist you in your quest to correctly identify heart rhythms.

1. **First and most important, look at your patient!** What is the patient's clinical picture, and how is it significant to the rhythm noted on the monitor?
2. Read EVERY strip from left to right, starting at the beginning of the strip.
3. Apply the five-step systematic approach that you will learn in this chapter.
4. Avoid shortcuts and assumptions. A quick glance at a strip will often lead to an incorrect interpretation.
5. Ask and answer each question in the five-step approach in the order that it is presented here. This is important for consistency.
6. You must master the accepted parameters for each dysrhythmia and then apply those parameters to each of the five steps when analyzing the strip.

THE FIVE-STEP APPROACH

There are several appropriate formats for EKG interpretation. The format that we have chosen follows a logical sequence in that we discuss EKG interpretation based first on heart rate and rhythm, followed by analysis of graphic representations of activities as they occur in the electrical conduction system of the heart.

This five-step approach, in order of application, includes analysis of the following:

Step 1:   Heart rate

Step 2:   Heart rhythm

Step 3:   P wave

Step 4:   PR Interval

Step 5:   QRS complex

EKG interpretation is more easily accomplished if each step is examined using this approach with each strip. Remember, quick glances can be deceiving.

Step 1: Heart Rate

Heart rate can be defined as the number of electrical impulses (as represented by PQRST complexes) conducted through the myocardium in 60 seconds (1 min). This analysis should be your first step in the interpretation of an EKG strip. When calculating heart rate, we usually are making reference to the **ventricular** heart rate. However, it is appropriate in certain strips to calculate both the **atrial** heart rate and the **ventricular** heart rate.

Simply stated, atrial heart rate can be determined by counting the number of P waves noted, while ventricular heart rate is determined by counting the number of QRS complexes. If atrial and ventricular heart rates are dissimilar, it is very important that you calculate both.

Recall now that the sinoatrial (SA) node discharges impulses at a rate of 60 to 100 times per minute. Therefore, a "normal" heart rate will be noted if the rate is calculated within a range of 60 to 100 beats per minute (BPM). If the rate is noted to be less than 60 beats per minute, we refer to this as **bradycardia.** In contrast, if the heart rate is greater than 100 beats per minute, the correct term is **tachycardia.** It is important to note here that these numbers are simply parameters or normal ranges to which we adhere when analyzing heart rate.

Keep in mind that your patient's clinical picture is critical to proper patient assessment and management. In other words, if your patient's heart rate is 58 beats per minute, he/she is technically bradycardic, based on the "normal" parameters. The patient's clinical picture, however, may indicate no evidence of hemodynamic compromise. Remember to ask yourself this question: "How is the rhythm significant to the patient's clinical picture?" Often you will find that a patient with a heart rate of 58 beats per minute is exhibiting no clinical symptomatology at all.

There are two common methods used to determine heart rate by visual examination of an EKG strip. The first and simplest way is called the **6-second method** (see Fig. 6-1). In order to properly use this method, you

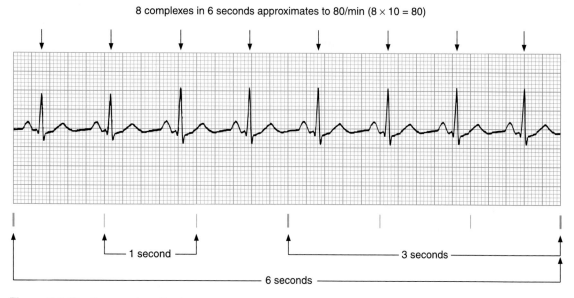

8 complexes in 6 seconds approximates to 80/min (8 × 10 = 80)

1 second

3 seconds

6 seconds

Figure 6-1 The 6-second method.

must first denote a 6-second interval on an EKG strip. Fortunately for us, EKG paper is commonly marked in either 3- or 6-second increments. Simply count the number of QRS complexes that occur within the 6-second interval and then multiply that number by 10. If the graph paper does not have 3- or 6-second marks, you can count the number of R waves in 30 large squares and multiply this number by 10. This will yield a close approximation of the patient's heart rate. This method is effective even when the rhythm is noted to be irregular.

The second common method used to determine heart rate by visual examination of an EKG strip is referred to as the **R-R interval** method. This method is most accurate if the heart rhythm is regular; otherwise it is only an estimation of heart rate. Recall from our discussion of EKG graph paper that there are 300 large boxes in a 60-second or 1-minute strip. With this in mind, you should look for a QRS complex (specifically an R wave) that falls on a heavy line on the strip. Then you should count the number of large boxes between the first R wave and the next R wave. After you determine that number, you then divide it into 300. For example, if there are 3 large boxes between two R waves, you would divide 3 into 300 and realize that the heart rate is 100 beats per minute (300 ÷ 3 = 100). Apply this method to the strip in Figure 6-2.

Remember that the "normal" heart rate is 60 to 100 beats per minute, below 60 beats per minute is a slow or bradycardic rate, and greater than 100 beats per minute is considered to be a fast or tachycardic rate. Heart rates can vary depending on many differing factors, including the general health of your patient, stress levels, strenuous exercise, or myocardial compromise. Again, you must constantly assess your patient while assessing his/her EKG strip.

Step 2: Heart Rhythm

Now we are ready to move on to Step 2 in the systematic approach to EKG analysis. Step 2 involves evaluating the rhythm of the heart. The term *rhythm* can be defined as the sequential beating of the heart as a result of the generation of electrical impulses. Synonyms for the word *rhythm* include *pattern, guide, model, order,* and *design.* Thus we can see that calculating the heart rhythm involves establishing a pattern of QRS complex occurrence.

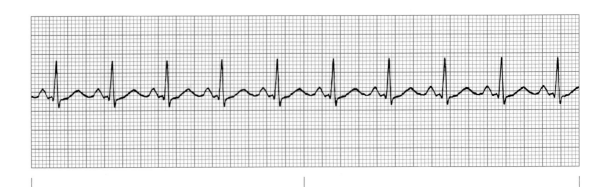

Figure 6-2 Normal sinus rhythm (rate of 100 BPM).

Heart rhythms are classified as either regular or irregular. Normally, the heart's rhythm is regular. To determine whether the ventricular rhythm is regular, you should measure the intervals between R waves. To determine whether the atrial rhythm is regular, you should measure the intervals between P waves. If the intervals vary by less than 0.06 second (or 1.5 small squares), the rhythm can be considered regular. If, however, the intervals are variable by greater than 0.06 second, the rhythm is considered to be irregular.

It may be helpful to use EKG calipers when you initially begin to analyze EKG rhythms. If calipers are not available, you may also measure intervals by making marks on a piece of paper placed on the EKG strip just below the peak of the R wave. After marking the area where each R wave occurred, look at the marks on your paper to identify a pattern. Then measure the distance between the marks with a ruler. If the marks are relatively equal distances apart, the rhythm is noted to be regular. If the distances between the marks vary noticeably, then the rhythm is probably irregular. Alterations of respiratory rate and depth may produce slight variations in heart rhythms.

Rhythms that are found to be irregular can be further classified as:

1. *Regularly irregular*—irregular rhythms that occur in a pattern
2. *Occasionally irregular*—only one or two R-R intervals are uneven
3. *Irregularly irregular*—R-R intervals exhibit no similarity

Regardless of whether the rhythm is regular or irregular, always remember to ask yourself that all-important question, "How is this rhythm clinically significant to my patient?"

Before moving on to Step 3, take a moment to review Steps 1 and 2.

Now look at the strips in Figures 6-3 and 6-4 and calculate the rate and rhythm of each one. After you think you have the answers, ask your instructor or tutor to verify your answers.

Step 3: The P Wave

First, let's recall the events that must occur to cause the formation of P waves on an EKG strip. We learned in Chapter 5 that the P wave is produced when the right and left atria depolarize. Depolarization of the atria is pro-

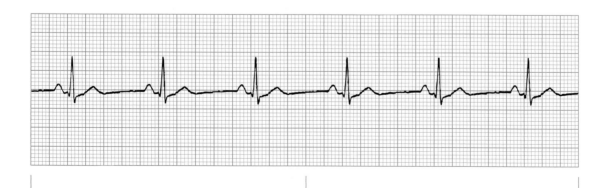

Figure 6-3 Practice strip for rate and rhythm analysis.

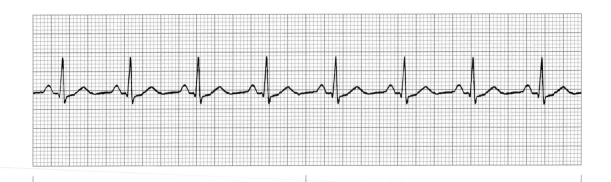

Figure 6-4 Practice strip for rate and rhythm analysis.

duced when an electrical impulse spreads throughout the atria via the internodal pathways. The P wave is noted as the first deviation from the isoelectric line on the EKG strip and should always be rounded and upright (positive) in limb Lead II. If the P wave is not upright in Lead II, you are not looking at a sinus rhythm (i.e., a rhythm that originated in the SA node).

There are five questions that should be asked when evaluating P waves:

1. Are P waves present?
2. Are the P waves occurring regularly?
3. Is there one P wave present for each QRS complex present?
4. Are the P waves smooth, rounded, and upright in appearance, or are they inverted?
5. Do all the P waves look similar?

Recall now that the SA node is the primary pacemaker of the heart and is located in the right atrium. If the SA node is pacing or firing at regular intervals, the P waves will also follow at regular intervals. This pattern would then be referred to as a *sinus rhythm*. In this text, the heart rhythms will be referenced according to their points of origin.

Step 4: The PR Interval

The PR Interval measures the time intervals from the onset of atrial contraction to the onset of ventricular contraction, or the time necessary for the electrical impulse to be conducted through the atria and the AV node. Although this component is called the PR Interval, it actually includes the entire P wave. The PR Interval is measured from the onset (or beginning) of the P wave to the onset of the Q wave of the QRS complex.

The normal length of the PR Interval is 0.12 to 0.20 second (3 to 5 small squares). The PR Interval should be constant across the EKG strip in order to be considered within normal limits. If the PR Interval is shortened (less than 0.12 sec), this may be an indication that the usual progression of the impulse is outside the normal route. Prolonged PR Intervals (greater than 0.20 sec) may indicate a delay in the electrical conduction pathway or an atrioventricular (AV) block.

There are three questions that should be asked when evaluating PR Intervals:

1. Are the PR Intervals greater than 0.20 second?
2. Are the PR Intervals less than 0.12 second?
3. Are the PR Intervals constant across the EKG strip?

Step 5: The QRS Complex

The QRS complex represents the depolarization (or contraction) of the ventricles. It is important to note whether all QRS complexes look alike, as this similarity will indicate that the electrical impulses are conducted in a consistent way.

The QRS complex is actually a group of waves, consisting of the:

Q wave   the first negative or downward deflection of this large complex. It is a small wave that precedes the R wave. Often the Q wave is not seen.

R wave   the first upward or positive deflection following the P wave. In chest Lead II, the R wave is the tallest waveform noted.

S wave   the sharp negative or downward deflection that follows the R wave.

You should refer now to Figure 6-5 in order to visualize the appearance of the QRS complex.

The overall appearance of the QRS, as well as its width, can provide important information about the electrical conduction system. When the electrical conduction system is functioning normally, the width of the QRS complex will be 0.12 second (3 small squares) or less (narrow). This nor-

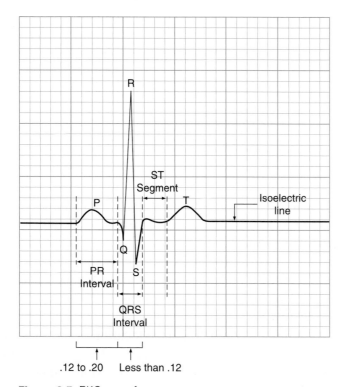

Figure 6-5 EKG waveforms.

mal or narrow QRS complex indicates that the impulse was not formed in the ventricles and is thus referred to as *supraventricular* or above the ventricles. Wide QRS complexes (greater than 0.12 sec or 3 small squares) indicate that the impulse is either of a ventricular origin or a supraventricular origin with aberrant (deviating from the normal course or pattern) conduction.

There are three questions that should be asked when evaluating QRS intervals:

1. Are QRS intervals greater than 0.12 second (wide)? If so, the complex may be ventricular in origin.
2. Are QRS intervals less than 0.12 second (narrow)? If so, the complex is most probably supraventricular in origin.
3. Are the QRS complexes similar in appearance across the EKG strip?

It is important to realize that the shape of QRS complexes will vary slightly in individual patients, depending on factors such as heart shape and size, health of the myocardium, and location and placement of electrodes.

THE 5 + 3 APPROACH

While it is imperative that you learn and remember the five basic steps to correctly interpret an EKG, we will now build on your knowledge in order to incorporate the correct interpretation of the 12-lead EKG strip. We call this approach the *5 + 3 approach*.

You will recall that the basic five steps include:

Rate	Rhythm	P wave	PR Interval	QRS complex

Now it's time to learn what we mean by the 5 + 3 approach:

Rate	Rhythm	P wave	PR Interval	QRS complex

PLUS

ST depression	ST elevation	Q wave

In order to learn each of the three new steps, we will look carefully at the ST segment as well as the Q wave. The ST segment begins with the end of the QRS complex and ends with the onset of the T wave. The normal ST segment is usually consistent with the isoelectric line of the EKG strip. It is during the period of the ST segment that ventricular repolarization is occurring. The point where the QRS complex meets the ST segment is commonly referred to as the *J point*.

Look now at Figure 6-5 and notice the location of the ST segment in the EKG. By visualizing the exact location of the ST segment, you will have a reference point as we discuss ST segment depression and elevation.

ST Segment Depression

ST segment depression occurs due to myocardial ischemia, secondary to myocardial tissue hypoxia (low level of oxygen). Hypoxia results in altered repolarization, which directly contributes to the development of ST segment depression. Significant ST segment depression is characterized by a dip below the isoelectric line of 1 to 2 millimeters or one to two small boxes on the EKG graph paper (see Fig. 6-6). The effect of hypoxia on repolarization may or may not produce inversion of the T wave. It is important to note and to reiterate that ST segment depression may be seen alone or with accompanying inversion of the T wave. As a rule, the larger the area of ischemic tissue, the more significant the EKG findings.

You as a health care provider must realize that appropriate and timely intervention is imperative if your patient is to receive the ultimate in quality patient care. Simply stated, if your index of suspicion is heightened by evidence of clinical and/or EKG findings, you must immediately administer 100% oxygen to the patient. Although there are many sophisticated, state-of-the-art equipment modalities available to today's health care provider, nothing—repeat, nothing—is more important than oxygen administration. This is especially true if your patient is complaining of chest pain and/or has a history of previous cardiac events.

Although the most common cause of ST segment depression is myocardial ischemia, you should understand that there are other causes. These include, but are not limited to:

- Ventricular hypertrophy
- Intraventricular conduction defects
- The medication digitalis (also commonly called Lanoxin or Digoxin)

Pathophysiologically, you should realize that the time when the patient's EKG strip demonstrates ST segment depression is one of the more critical times to strive for reversal of the myocardial ischemia. At this point there is no irreversible injury to the myocardium. As we proceed through the subsequent chapters of this textbook, you will often see the phrase **Time Is Muscle** or **Time Is Myocardium.** The more literal interpretation of this phrase simply says to you, the health care provider, that the criticality of

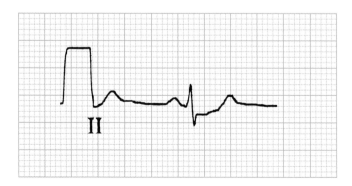

Figure 6-6 ST segment depression.

immediate oxygen administration cannot be overemphasized. The patient's outcome may quite literally depend on it. The longer **time** it takes for intervention to occur, the greater the possibility of irreparable **muscle** damage.

ST Segment Elevation

Our reference to ST segment elevation will presume that the patient did not receive the necessary oxygen in a timely and appropriate manner. Thus the succession from hypoxia to ischemia to injury will progress. At this point, the ST segment will become elevated. Significant ST segment elevation is characterized by a rise above the isoelectric line of 1 to 2 millimeters or one to two small boxes on the EKG graph paper (see Fig. 6-7).

The most common cause of ST segment elevation is myocardial injury secondary to acute myocardial infarction (MI). Other causes may include:

- Coronary artery vasospasm (Prinzmetal's angina)
- Pericarditis (EKG evidence is usually present in all leads)
- Ventricular aneurysm
- Early repolarization (in young children)

As a general rule, ST segment elevation will occur within the first 1 to 2 hours after the onset of myocardial hypoxia, if the patient is not properly managed. At this point, we must remind you that IT IS NOT TOO LATE to

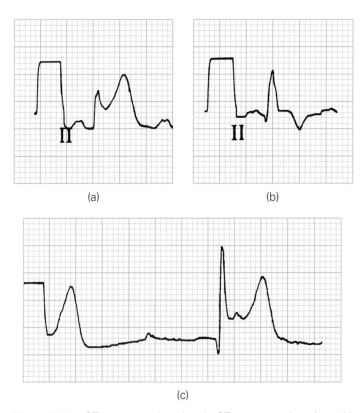

(a)   (b)

(c)

Figure 6-7 a: ST segment elevation. b: ST segment elevation with T wave inversion. c: ST segment elevation with tall T wave.

TABLE 6-1 MYOCARDIAL TISSUE HYPOXIA: EARLY TREATMENT MEASURES	
Basic Interventions	Advanced Interventions
Calm and reassure patient	Administer oxygen
Administer oxygen	Initiate cardiac monitoring
Prehospital—notify advanced life support (ALS) backup (as indicated)	Obtain a 12-lead EKG; establish an intravenous (IV) lifeline

intercede. Although the myocardial hypoxia is showing signs of progression, the tissue damage at this point is not irreparable. Thus, early intervention and appropriate management are critical to your patient's outcome. Early intervention includes, but is not limited to, the interventions shown in Table 6-1.

PATHOLOGIC Q WAVES

The development of the **pathologic Q wave** indicates irreversible tissue damage, or death of the myocardial tissue. A pathologic Q wave is defined as a width greater than or equal to one small box (1 mm) or a depth greater than one-third of the R wave in the same lead. Following myocardial infarction and inadequate intervention, and as a result of the absence of depolarization current from dead myocardial tissue, a deep Q wave may be seen.

The appearance of a pathologic Q wave is an ominous sign and most commonly indicates a more discouraging patient outcome. This is true because at this point myocardial tissue damage has occurred and may be significant. After several months, fibrous scarring will replace the infarcted tissue. The presence of scar tissue in and around the myocardium may hamper the heart's mechanical and/or electrical activity.

Figure 6-8 shows the EKG changes that occur at each stage of an MI; Figure 6-9 shows a normal 12-lead EKG for comparison.

You must understand that, when considering the 5 + 3 approach, the final three steps must be carefully considered. It is imperative to your understanding of 12-lead EKG interpretation that you note the evidence (or the lack thereof) of each of the steps. In other words, ask yourself the questions:

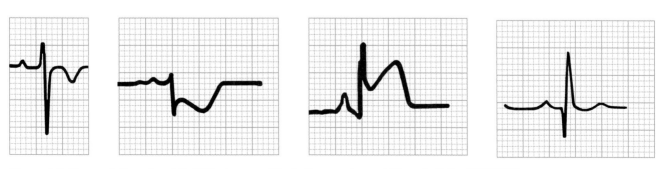

Figure 6-8 The evolution of an MI: EKG changes. (Illustration courtesy of Ricaurte Solís, NREMT-P.)

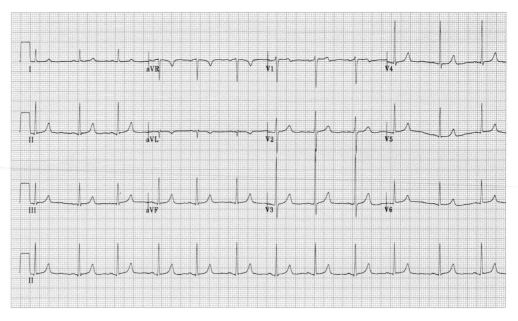

Figure 6-9 Normal 12-lead EKG.

1. "Is there evidence of ST segment depression, and if so, in which leads does it appear?"

2. "Is there evidence of ST segment elevation, and if so, in which leads does it occur?"

3. "Is there evidence of Q waves, in which leads do the Q waves appear, and are the Q waves pathologic or nonpathologic?"

You should be aware that evidence in each of the +3 steps may not be present. In other words, an EKG may demonstrate ST segment depression, ST segment elevation, and pathologic Q waves in previously specified leads, allowing you to unequivocally identify a specific type of myocardial infarction. However, a single finding in one step of the +3 approach may also be indicative of an early MI. A clear example could be the presence of ST segment depression in a specific lead group, with no other findings in the +3 approach.

Assessment of the patient's clinical presentation (i.e., signs and symptoms) is critical in determining the presence of an acute myocardial infarction. In addition, you must remember that EKG changes that are the most indicative of the presence of an acute myocardial infarction include ST segment elevation and presence of a pathologic Q wave. Recall the important point that **Time Is Muscle,** and act accordingly.

REVIEW QUESTIONS: CHAPTER 6

1. The sinoatrial node is located in the:

    a. Right atrium

    b. Right ventricle

    c. Purkinje fiber tract

    d. Atrioventricular septum

2. The intrinsic firing rate of the AV node is:

   a. 15–25 BPM

   b. 25–35 BPM

   c. 35–45 BPM

   d. 40–60 BPM

3. The intrinsic firing rate of the SA node in the adult is:

   a. 20–60 BPM

   b. 40–80 BPM

   c. 60–100 BPM

   d. 80–100 BPM

4. The 12-lead electrocardiogram is used to evaluate all of the following except:

   a. Pulse rate

   b. Valvular dysfunction

   c. Electrical activity in the heart

   d. Isolate waveforms indicative of AMI

5. The PR Interval should normally be _____ or smaller.

   a. 0.10 sec

   b. 0.12 sec

   c. 0.08 sec

   d. 0.20 sec

6. The QRS interval should normally be _____ or smaller.

   a. 0.20 sec

   b. 0.12 sec

   c. 0.18 sec

   d. 0.36 sec

7. ST segment depression indicates:

   a. Myocardial ischemia

   b. Coronary vasospasm

   c. Prinzmetal's angina

   d. Chronic pericarditis

8. The QRS complex is produced when the:

   a. Ventricles repolarize

   b. Ventricles depolarize

   c. Ventricles contract

   d. Both b and c

9. The normal conduction pattern of the heart follows:

    1. SA node

    2. Purkinje fibers

    3. Bundle of His

    4. AV node

    5. Bundle branches

    6. Internodal pathways

    a. 1, 5, 2, 4, 6, 3

    b. 1, 6, 4, 3, 5, 2

    c. 1, 4, 3, 6, 5, 2

    d. 1, 2, 3, 4, 5, 6

10. ST segment elevation is a primary indicator of:

    a. Ventricular atrophy

    b. Ventricular hypertrophy

    c. Myocardial injury

    d. Atrial aneurysm

11. The T wave on the EKG strip represents:

    a. Rest period

    b. Bundle of His

    c. Atrial contraction

    d. Ventricular contraction

12. When interpreting dysrhythmias, you should remember that the most important key is the:

    a. PR Interval

    b. Rate and rhythm

    c. Presence of dysrhythmias

    d. Patient's clinical appearance

7

ACUTE MYOCARDIAL INFARCTIONS

Objectives

Upon completion of this chapter, the student will be able to:

1. Discuss the anatomy of the coronary arteries and the coronary veins

2. Discuss guidelines for differentiating angina pectoris from acute myocardial infarction based on:
   a. Clinical presentation
   b. EKG findings

3. Discuss chest pain based on:
   a. Signs and symptoms
   b. Standard treatment modalities

4. Review the clinical significance of acute myocardial infarction (AMI)

Cardiac emergencies, including acute myocardial infarctions, continue to be one of the nation's leading causes of death. Heart attacks and other cardiac emergencies affect more than 5 million individuals each year, and more than 1 million deaths each year are directly attributed to heart disease. Your understanding of 12-lead EKGs will enhance your ability to assess and treat the patient who presents with chest pain in a more time-efficient manner.

CORONARY ARTERY ANATOMY

Understanding the structure and functions of the coronary arteries and the coronary sinus is a critical component of 12-lead EKG interpretation.

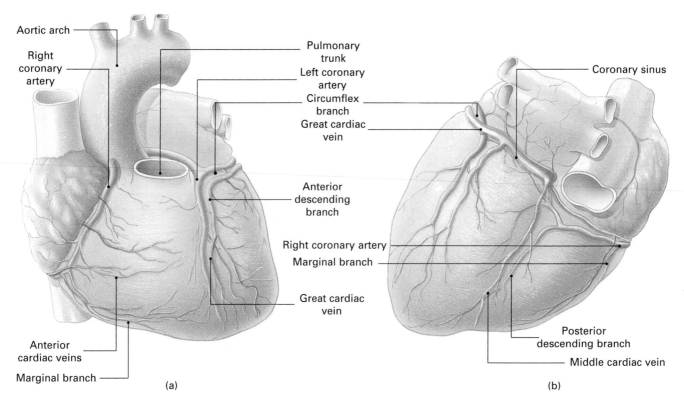

Figure 7-1 Coronary circulation.

The importance of these structures will be reviewed and emphasized in this chapter.

The right and left coronary arteries arise and branch off from the proximal portion of the aorta and function to transport oxygenated blood throughout the heart muscle (myocardium). The coronary vessels receive their blood supply during ventricular diastole (relaxation). Figure 7-1 depicts the coronary circulation. Table 7-1 gives the divisions or branches of the coronary arteries; Table 7-2 shows the distribution of blood supply to the myocardium.

There are two main branches of the coronary arteries that are located on the surface of the heart. Usually smaller than the left coronary artery, the right coronary artery does not supply as large a portion of the heart muscle with blood as does the left coronary artery. It should be noted that there is a significant degree of individual variance in the normal coronary artery distribution. It is from these important structures that blood is supplied to the myocardial tissues by way of small penetrating arterioles.

TABLE 7-1 CORONARY ARTERY DIVISIONS/BRANCHES	
Left Coronary Arteries	Right Coronary Arteries
Left anterior descending	Posterior descending
Marginal	Marginal
Circumflex	

TABLE 7-2 DISTRIBUTION OF BLOOD SUPPLY TO THE MYOCARDIUM

Left Coronary Arteries	Right Coronary Arteries
Anterior left ventricular wall	Lateral wall of the right ventricle
Lateral wall of the left ventricle	A portion of the electrical conduction system
Posterior wall of the left ventricle	Posterior wall of left ventricle
Left interventricular septal wall	Inferior wall of left ventricle

The Left Coronary Artery

As the left coronary artery leaves the aorta, it immediately divides into the left anterior descending artery and the circumflex artery. The anterior descending artery is the major branch of the left coronary artery and supplies blood to most of the anterior part of the heart. A marginal branch of the left coronary artery supplies blood to the lateral wall of the left ventricle. The circumflex branch of the left coronary artery extends around to the posterior side of the heart and its branches supply blood to much of the posterior wall of the heart. Each of these divisions has numerous branches that form a network of blood vessels.

The Right Coronary Artery

The right coronary artery extends from the aorta around to the posterior part of the heart. Branches of the right coronary artery supply blood to the lateral wall of the right ventricle. A branch of the right coronary artery called the posterior interventricular artery or posterior descending artery lies in the posterior interventricular region and supplies blood to the posterior and inferior part of the heart's left ventricle. The right coronary artery branches also supply oxygen-rich blood to a portion of the electrical conduction system.

Collateral circulation allows for an alternate path of blood flow in the event of vascular occlusion and is a protective mechanism. Numerous **anastomoses** (communications between two or more vessels) between various branches of the coronary arteries allow for collateral circulation. The body's innate ability to develop collateral circulation enables select individuals to compensate for atherosclerotic deposits in their coronary arteries, thereby allowing them to remain virtually asymptomatic for extended periods.

THE CORONARY SINUS (GREAT CARDIAC VEIN)

Draining the myocardial tissue on the left side of the heart is the **great cardiac vein.** A smaller cardiac vein drains the right margin of the heart. Toward the posterior part of the coronary sulcus (ditch), these veins converge and empty into a large venous cavity called the **coronary sinus.** The coronary sinus is a short trunk that serves to receive deoxygenated blood from the major veins of the myocardium. This trunk empties into the right atrium. The coronary veins roughly correspond positionally with the coronary arteries throughout the myocardium.

Now that we have reviewed the anatomy of the coronary circulation, we will discuss various pathologies that result from coronary insufficiency.

ANGINA PECTORIS

Angina pectoris is described as pain that results from a reduction in blood supply to myocardial tissue. The pain is typically temporary. If blood flow is quickly restored, little or no permanent change or damage may result. Angina is characterized by chest pain or discomfort deep in the sternal area and is often described as heaviness, pressure, or moderately severe pain. It is quite often mistaken for indigestion. This pain can be referred to the neck, lower jaw, or left shoulder, arm, and fingers.

Angina pectoris most often results from narrowed and/or hardened coronary arterial walls. The reduced blood flow results in a reduced supply of oxygen to cardiac muscle cells. The pain is often predictably associated with exercise, due to the increased pumping activity of the heart, which requires more oxygen than the narrowed blood vessels can supply.

Frequently, angina pectoris is relieved by rest and medications such as nitroglycerin. Nitroglycerin causes blood vessel dilation, which consequently reduces the workload of the heart, thus reducing the need for oxygen because the heart has to pump blood against a lesser pressure. The blood tends to remain in the dilated blood vessels, and less blood is returned to the heart for distribution.

ACUTE MYOCARDIAL INFARCTIONS

An acute myocardial infarction results from a prolonged lack of blood flow to a portion of the myocardial tissue that leads to a lack of oxygen. Eventually, myocardial cellular death will follow. Myocardial infarctions (MIs) vary with the amount of myocardial tissue and the portion of the heart that is affected. If blood supply to cardiac muscle is reestablished within 10 to 20 minutes, there will usually be no permanent injury. If oxygen deprivation lasts longer, cellular death will result. Within 30 to 60 seconds after blockage of a coronary blood vessel, functional changes become evident. The electrical properties of the cardiac muscle are altered and the ability of the cardiac muscle to function properly is lost.

The most common cause of myocardial infarctions is thrombus formation that blocks a coronary artery. Coronary arteries narrowed by atherosclerotic damage provide one of the conditions that increase the likelihood of myocardial infarction. Atherosclerotic lesions partially block blood vessels, resulting in disorderly blood flow due to the rough surfaces of the lesions. These changes increase the probability of thrombus formation.

Signs and symptoms of an acute myocardial infarction may be quite similar to those of angina pectoris. Clear differences include that the pain caused by an AMI lasts longer and is usually not relieved by rest (see Table 7-3).

TABLE 7-3 DIFFERENTIAL SYMPTOMOLOGY: ANGINA VERSUS AMI

Signs/Symptoms—Angina Pectoris	Signs/Symptoms—Acute Myocardial Infarction
Chest pain is of short duration—usually lasts 3–10 min; usually relieved by nitroglycerin	Chest pain usually lasts more than 2 hr; not relieved by nitroglycerin
Brought on by stress or exercise and relieved by rest	Usually not precipitated by exercise or stress; not relieved by rest
May be accompanied by dysrhythmias	Usually accompanied by dysrhythmias
Patient usually do not have nausea, vomiting, or diaphoresis	Patients commonly complain of nausea and vomiting and are often profoundly diaphoretic

CHEST PAIN

Cardiac versus Noncardiac

Chest pain of cardiac origin may present in various ways. As discussed previously in this chapter, this type of chest pain may be indicative of serious illness, myocardial ischemia, or myocardial injury, or may simply indicate stress or exercise-related hypoxia.

Chest pain is the most common presenting symptom of cardiac disease, as well as the most common patient complaint. Chest pain of cardiac origin is typically described as crushing or squeezing in nature and is commonly associated with nausea, vomiting, and diaphoresis (profuse sweating). The pain is often located substernally and may radiate to the jaw(s), shoulder(s), arm(s), and finger(s).

Chest pain from an acute myocardial infarction may escalate in intensity. Patients may express a feeling of impending doom and may exhibit extreme anxiety. A common obstacle to timely intervention by the health care provider when dealing with a patient who complains of chest pain is denial. Patients often deny the possibility that they may indeed be experiencing a heart attack, with thoughts such as, "It can't happen to me." Often patients prefer to believe that they are merely experiencing indigestion and that these symptoms will be gone by morning. Unfortunately it may be the patient, rather than the symptoms, who is gone by morning! With proper public education, many lives have been saved that otherwise would have been lost; this is due in large part to the simple fact that many thousands of laypersons have been certified in the skill of cardiopulmonary resuscitation (CPR).

It should be noted that, in special circumstances, patients may experience no chest pain at all and still have sustained a myocardial infarction. This is true primarily in the diabetic patient with advanced neuropathy, due to destruction of nerve endings and thus the inability to perceive pain. The scenario with which diabetic patients may present is often congestive heart failure. Some elderly patients may experience an AMI without chest pain; most commonly their only presenting symptom will be the complaint of profound weakness.

Standard Treatment Modalities for Cardiac-Related Chest Pain

The goal of management of the patient with symptomatic chest pain is to strive to interrupt the infarction process. This can be achieved through interventions such as immediate and effective oxygen administration, pain alleviation, management of dysrhythmias, and possibly initiation of thrombolytic therapy in order to limit the progression of the infarct.

Without a doubt, the most important drug any patient with chest pain can receive is oxygen. Time and again, in this and other textbooks, you will see that statement—simply because it is true and it is critically important to the viability of your patient. Other considerations regarding treatment include:

- Administering 100% oxygen
- Establishing an intravenous (IV) lifeline (according to local protocols)
- Measuring oxygen saturation level (pulse oximetry), if equipment is available
- Performing continuous cardiac monitoring; obtain 12-lead EKG
- Providing pain control and management (i.e., nitroglycerin, morphine sulfate, Demerol, etc.) (according to local protocols)
- Initiating thrombolytic therapy/aspirin

Remember that the focus of assessment and treatment of the patient who presents with chest pain centers on the immediate oxygenation of hypoxic tissue. Treatment initiatives will vary depending upon your patient's specific situation; however, you must focus on continual and thorough assessment until such time as the patient is clinically stable.

Noncardiac Causes of Chest Pain

Causes of noncardiac chest pain are numerous. However, remember that chest pain is cardiac in nature until proven otherwise, especially in the prehospital arena. Some of the causes of noncardiac chest pain include, but are not limited to, the following:

- *Pleurisy*—inflammation of the covering of the lungs (pleura)
- *Costrochondritis*—inflammation of intercostal muscles (located between the ribs)
- *Pericarditis*—inflammation of the pericardial sac (surrounding the heart)
- *Myocardial contusion*—secondary to chest trauma (high incidence of dysrhythmias)
- *Muscle strain*—secondary to overstretching of the chest wall muscles
- *Trauma*—secondary to injury to the chest wall and/or organs contained within the chest

Examples of chest injuries secondary to trauma include:

- *Hemothorax*—collection of blood within the pleural cavity
- *Pneumothorax*—collection of air within the pleural cavity
- *Hemopneumothorax*—collection of blood and air within the pleural cavity
- *Tension pneumothorax*—air trapped in the thoracic cavity without an escape route; pressure builds and affects the lungs, heart, and other vital organs

Chest trauma can produce severe chest pain and may indicate a serious condition that requires immediate intervention. Any patient who exhibits chest pain, regardless of the clinical presentation, should be monitored for the possible occurrence of dysrhythmias. Remember the old adage about an ounce of prevention? When dealing with chest pain, this adage definitely applies, because . . . **Time Is Muscle!**

CLINICAL SIGNIFICANCE OF ACUTE MYOCARDIAL INFARCTIONS

As mentioned at the beginning of this chapter, cardiac emergencies, including acute myocardial infarctions, continue to be one of the nation's leading causes of death. Thus the significance of the patient's condition, as well as the need for early intervention for patients with suspected AMI, is paramount. An acute myocardial infarction may be a staggering event involving electrical conduction system disturbances as well as mechanical failure secondary to infarcted tissue.

PATIENT ASSESSMENT

Recall now that **Time Is Muscle** and act accordingly. Thus, timely assessment and management, including immediate oxygen administration, must be rapidly initiated and completed within a 10-minute time interval. Your initial assessment and evaluation should focus on the patient's general appearance. You will probably note that patients who are suffering from an AMI will tend to remain quiet and still. These patients also tend to prefer a sitting position. The Fowler's or semi-Fowler's position tends to allow the patient to breathe more comfortably and may decrease the workload of the myocardium.

A thorough and timely evaluation and management of the patient's ABCs is imperative. Any problem encountered during this evaluation must be managed quickly, followed by a rapid assessment of the vital signs. Because of the wide variations of the presenting vital signs, the clinician should be aware that vital signs are not necessarily reliable in diagnosing an AMI. In spite of this fact, it is important that you monitor and record these signs at frequent intervals.

One of the most important assessment tools that you will utilize when managing the suspected AMI patient is the cardiac monitor. Dysrhythmias that originate from ischemic and injured myocardial tissues are a common complication of acute myocardial infarctions. It is critical that you understand that in the clinical setting, dysrhythmias may simply be warning signs or they may signal severe, life-threatening events. In either case, you must not ignore the presence of any abnormal heart rhythm when dealing with a patient who exhibits the textbook clinical presentation of an acute myocardial infarction. Although the 3-lead EKG strip will adequately depict the heart rate and rhythm, the 12-lead EKG has the ability to afford a comprehensive picture of the myocardial events occurring during an acute myocardial infarction.

In the prehospital arena, your suspicion of an acute myocardial infarction must be based on a combination of a positive 12-lead EKG and the patient's clinical picture (signs and symptoms). In the in-hospital setting, these two factors in addition to serum enzyme changes and the development of pathologic Q waves will further assist in your conclusion. Keep in mind, however, that a negative 12-lead EKG does NOT rule out the presence of an AMI. Remember also that any patient who complains of chest pain must be thoroughly evaluated and that management of the patient should continue until the possibility of AMI is ruled out by the physician.

REVIEW QUESTIONS: CHAPTER 7

1. The right and left coronary arteries branch off of the:
    a. Ventricular artery
    b. Myocardial sulcus
    c. Proximal portion of the aorta
    d. Distal portion of the aorta

2. Collateral circulation allows for:
    a. Alternate path of blood flow in the event of occlusion
    b. Circulation continuum during diastole
    c. Maintaining artery patency during spasms
    d. Blood flow continuum during systole

3. The pain of angina pectoris:
    a. Is always constant
    b. Is typically temporary
    c. Occurs only during rest
    d. Is never mistaken for indigestion

4. Myocardial infarction is:
    a. Always temporary
    b. Usually diagnosed within 24 hr
    c. Age limited in most patients
    d. Due to myocardial cell death

5. The most common cause of AMIs is:

   a. Coronary vasospasms

   b. Atherosclerotic lesions

   c. Thrombus formation

   d. Arteriosclerotic blebs

6. In acute myocardial infarctions, chest pain is:

   a. Short in duration and relieved by nitroglycerin

   b. Short in duration but not relieved by nitroglycerin

   c. Long in duration and relieved by nitroglycerin

   d. Long in duration and not relieved by nitroglycerin

7. Patients experiencing an acute myocardial infarction will always complain of chest pain.

   a. True

   b. False

8. ST segment elevation is a primary indicator of:

   a. Ventricular atrophy

   b. Ventricular hypertrophy

   c. Myocardial injury

   d. Atrial aneurysm

9. The T wave on the EKG strip represents:

   a. Rest period

   b. Bundle of His

   c. Atrial contraction

   d. Ventricular contraction

10. When interpreting dysrhythmias, you should remember that the most important key is the:

    a. PR Interval

    b. Rate and rhythm

    c. Presence of dysrhythmias

    d. Patient's clinical appearance

11. The primary goal of management of the patient with symptomatic chest pain is to:

    a. Interrupt the infarction process

    b. Augment the infarction process

    c. Institute thrombolytic therapy

    d. Increase myocardial oxygen consumption

12. Management of a patient who is suspected of having sustained a myocardial contusion should:

   a. Focus primarily on the associated and isolated chest injury

   b. Be similar to the treatment administered to a suspected MI patient

   c. Only be initiated at the definitive care facility following transport

   d. Be completed in the prehospital arena, prior to transport to the hospital

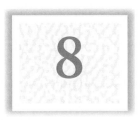

8

MYOCARDIAL ISCHEMIA, INJURY, AND NECROSIS

Objectives

Upon completion of this chapter, the student will be able to:

1. Describe the importance of timely treatment and transport of a patient with a suspected acute myocardial infarction (AMI).

2. Define myocardial ischemia, injury, and necrosis

3. Discuss myocardial ischemia, including:
   a. signs and symptoms
   b. EKG changes

4. Discuss myocardial injury, including:
   a. signs and symptoms
   b. EKG changes

5. Discuss myocardial infarction (necrosis), including:
   a. signs and symptoms
   b. EKG changes

6. Review the clinical significance of myocardial ischemia, injury, and necrosis

Time Is Muscle is a phrase that is used worldwide to indicate the importance of timely intervention in a scenario wherein the patient is suspected to be experiencing an acute myocardial infarction. The less time it takes to start definitive treatment, the less muscle will be lost. Conversely, this axiom can be viewed as follows: the more time it takes to start definitive treatment, the more myocardial muscle is lost. This chapter will focus on the changes that occur at the cellular level as a result of oxygen deprivation. In addition, we will discuss specific EKG changes that can be anticipated as a result of myocardial ischemia, myocardial injury, and necrosis of the myocardial tissues.

TIME IS MUSCLE (MYOCARDIUM)

As stated in Chapter 7, the fundamental goal of management of the patient with symptomatic chest pain is to strive to interrupt the infarction process. It is important to reiterate that this can be achieved through interventions such as appropriate oxygen administration, pain management, and recognition and treatment of dysrhythmias. Based on standard inclusion/exclusion criteria and local protocol, thrombolytic therapy may be in order to limit the progression of the infarct. As repeatedly stated, the most important drug that any patient with chest pain can receive is oxygen. Time and again, in this and other textbooks, you will see this statement—simply because it is true and it is critically important to your patient's outcome.

Again, and at the risk of being redundant, we feel it is critical that you remember that the focus of assessment and treatment of the patient who presents with chest pain centers on the immediate oxygenation of hypoxic tissue. Treatment initiatives will vary depending upon your patient's specific situation; however, you must focus on continual and thorough assessment until such time as the patient is clinically stable.

INFARCT REGIONS AND DEFINITIONS

Typically, the damage caused by an acute myocardial infarction evolves into three distinct sectors (see Fig. 8-1). From outside to inside, these sectors include the ischemic area, the injured area, and the infarcted area.

Myocardial ischemia deprivation of oxygen and other nutrients to the heart muscle (myocardium); tendency to produce repolarization abnormalities

Myocardial injury injury (damage) to the heart muscle (myocardium); most commonly results from and follows myocardial ischemia

Myocardial necrosis death of the myocardial tissue (myocardial infarction)

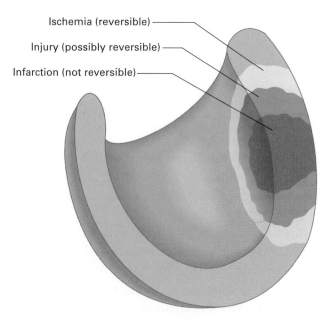

Ischemia (reversible)
Injury (possibly reversible)
Infarction (not reversible)

Figure 8-1 Sectors of damage from myocardial infarction (MI).

Myocardial Ischemia

Myocardial ischemia may also be defined as:

- A temporary shortage of oxygen at the cellular level

OR

- A transient absence of blood supply to the myocardial tissues

Whichever definition you prefer to learn, the most substantive point that you must learn and understand is that the lack of or absence of oxygen to the myocardial cells can be, if left uncorrected, a life-altering event.

Ischemic changes cause a delay in the depolarization and repolarization of the cells around the area of infarct. The human body reacts to this event by perceiving chest pain. In addition, other signs and symptoms indicative of myocardial ischemia may include fatigue, diaphoresis, and varying degrees of anxiety. Once proper intervention has transpired and the return of adequate blood flow and reoxygenation is accomplished, the pain typically goes away and the myocardial cells return to a normal or near normal state.

EKG changes with myocardial ischemia include ST segment depression, T wave inversion, or peaked T waves (see Fig. 8-2). The most significant and frequently identifiable of these EKG changes is ST segment depression, which usually occurs in two or more contiguous leads. In order to be diagnostic, the ST segment depression should be at least 1 millimeter or 0.08 second (2 small boxes) below the isoelectric line, with calculation initiating at the J point. You should recall that the J point is the point on the EKG strip where the QRS complex meets the ST segment. ST segment depression typically reverts to normal following the administration of oxygen if this intervention corrects the myocardial hypoxia. ST segment depression may be evident on a 12-lead EKG strip following both angina and strenuous exercise.

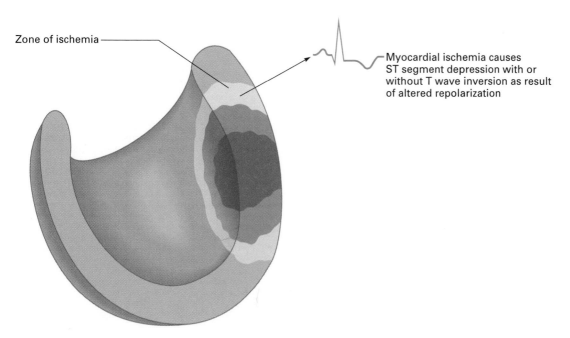

Zone of ischemia

Myocardial ischemia causes ST segment depression with or without T wave inversion as result of altered repolarization

Figure 8-2 EKG changes reflecting myocardial ischemia.

Myocardial Injury

In the important concept that **Time Is Muscle,** the continuum of the hypoxic state of the myocardial cells will cause progression to myocardial injury. At this time in the event, the injured cells are still viable and salvageable; however, the cells will die if the hypoxic state is not quickly alleviated. Myocardial injury can be extensive enough to produce a decrease in electrical conduction and/or pump (mechanical) function.

Without appropriate intervention, at this point in the myocardial event, the patient's signs and symptoms may intensify slightly. In addition to the signs and symptoms listed previously, the patient may continue to complain of chest pain of increased magnitude. Clinically you may note that the patient becomes pale and his/her anxiety level may increase. In addition, it is at this point that some patients may begin to complain of dyspnea (difficulty in breathing).

EKG changes with myocardial injury include ST segment elevation and/or T wave inversion (see Fig. 8-3). The most significant and frequently identifiable of these EKG changes is ST segment elevation, which usually occurs in two or more contiguous leads. In order to be diagnostic, the ST segment elevation should be at least 1 millimeter or 0.08 second (2 small boxes) above the isoelectric line, with calculation initiating at the J point.

ST segment elevation provides the primary indication of myocardial injury in progress. There may also be T wave inversion suggestive of the presence of ischemia. ST segments are elevated in the leads that represent the area of injury and may be depressed in the opposite leads.

Myocardial Necrosis

As the myocardial ischemia and injury continue uncorrected, some cells begin to sustain irreversible damage and infarct. At this point, cellular death

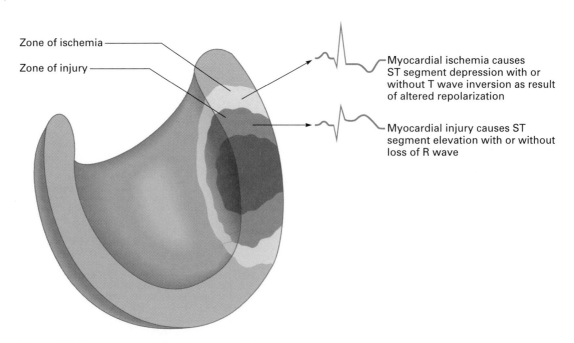

Zone of ischemia

Zone of injury

Myocardial ischemia causes ST segment depression with or without T wave inversion as result of altered repolarization

Myocardial injury causes ST segment elevation with or without loss of R wave

Figure 8-3 EKG changes reflecting myocardial injury.

(necrosis) occurs and the patient experiences a myocardial infarction. It is critical at this point that you, the health care provider, realize that, at the point of myocardial necrosis, the myocardial tissue and cells will not—CANNOT—return to normal, even when reoxygenation is initiated. The necrotic cells become scar tissue and do not respond to electrical stimulus or provide any contractile functions. This is the point that we must strive not to allow the patient to reach. Now you may better comprehend the concept of **Time Is Muscle!**

Signs and symptoms of an acute myocardial infarction are numerous. Recall that the precipitating event of an AMI is often a thrombus. As discussed in detail in Chapter 7, the most common presenting sign or symptom of AMI is substernal or epigastric chest pain. Other common signs and symptoms include diaphoresis, anxiety, dyspnea, nausea, vomiting, pallor, general weakness, and malaise. As a health care provider, you should be aware that some patients who are experiencing an AMI will express a feeling of impending doom. You are well advised, if a patient tells you that he/she is going to die, to believe the patient . . . many times he/she will do just that!

The development of the pathologic Q waves often begins within the first 2 hours after the MI and, in most cases, is complete within 24 hours. One of the more reliable EKG changes noted when a patient is experiencing an AMI is the presence of pathologic Q waves (see Fig. 8-4). However, you should realize that the appearance of the pathologic Q wave is a later finding than is the development of ST segment elevation.

A Q wave is considered abnormal if it is equal or greater than 0.04 second (1 small box) in width and has a depth of 25% or more of the height of the succeeding R wave. We should remind you that the size of the pathologic Q wave depends upon the degree of infarct that the myocardial mus-

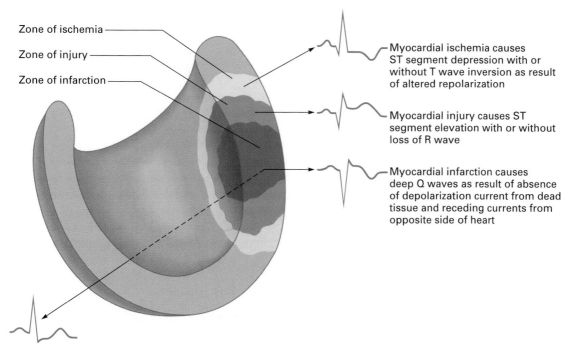

Zone of ischemia

Zone of injury

Zone of infarction

Myocardial ischemia causes ST segment depression with or without T wave inversion as result of altered repolarization

Myocardial injury causes ST segment elevation with or without loss of R wave

Myocardial infarction causes deep Q waves as result of absence of depolarization current from dead tissue and receding currents from opposite side of heart

Figure 8-4 EKG changes reflecting myocardial infarct.

cle has sustained. If damage is very minimal, the pathologic Q wave may not develop. There are also non–Q wave MIs, which we will discuss in a later chapter.

CLINICAL SIGNIFICANCE OF MYOCARDIAL ISCHEMIA, INJURY, AND NECROSIS

As emphasized in Chapter 7, all chest pain is considered clinically significant and thus must be managed in a timely and appropriate manner. Although we are not expected to definitively diagnose an acute myocardial infarction in the prehospital arena, or in the emergency department (ED) or intensive care unit (ICU) for that matter, it is critically important that we learn and commit to memory the various signs and symptoms that will be exhibited as the patient progresses from myocardial ischemia through the myocardial injury event and finally (without proper intervention) into the myocardial necrotic state.

Thus timely assessment and management, including immediate oxygen administration, must be rapidly initiated and completed within a 10-minute time interval. Your initial assessment and evaluation should focus on the patient's general appearance. Remember that **Time Is Muscle,** and act accordingly.

REVIEW QUESTIONS: CHAPTER 8

1. The coronary arteries receive oxygenated blood from the:
   a. Aorta
   b. Coronary sinus
   c. Pulmonary veins
   d. Pulmonary arteries

2. Signs and symptoms the health care provider may expect to observe in a patient with necrotic heart tissue could include:
   a. Dysrhythmias
   b. Congestive heart failure
   c. Cardiogenic shock (severe)
   d. All of the above are possible

3. The function of the chordae tendineae and papillary muscles is to:
   a. Prevent backflow of blood into the ventricles
   b. Protect the coronary orifices when the aortic valve opens
   c. Prevent backflow of blood into the atrium
   d. Facilitate backflow of blood from the aorta

4. The right atrium receives blood from the myocardium via the:
   a. Left marginal branch

b. Inferior vena cava

c. Great cardiac vein

d. Internal carotid artery

5. The coronary sinus returns deoxygenated blood from the:

a. Aorta

b. Myocardium

c. Pulmonary veins

d. Pulmonary arteries

6. Most cardiac dysrhythmias are caused by ischemia secondary to hypoxia; therefore the most appropriate drug to give a patient with any dysrhythmia is:

a. Oxygen

b. D5W

c. Lidocaine

d. Morphine

7. Defined as death of the myocardial tissue, myocardial infarction commonly results from:

a. Myocardial necrosis

b. Myocardial injury

c. Myocardial ischemia

d. Muscle oxygenation

8. EKG changes that may be anticipated as a result of myocardial ischemia, injury, and/or necrosis of the myocardial tissues include all of the following except:

a. PR Interval prolongation

b. ST segment elevation

c. ST segment depression

d. Pathologic Q wave

9. The development of the pathologic Q waves often begins within the first 2 hours after the MI, and in most cases is complete within:

a. 60 min

b. 30 min

c. 24 hr

d. 48 hr

10. ST segment depression may be evident on a 12-lead EKG strip following both angina and strenuous exercise.

a. False

b. True

11. EKG changes of significance with myocardial ischemia include ST segment depression, T wave inversion, or:

a. Depressed T wave

b. Peaked T wave

c. Peaked P wave

d. Inverted P wave

12. Chest pain should be considered to be cardiac in origin and managed accordingly until proven otherwise.

a. True

b. False

9

INTERPRETATION OF INFERIOR MIs

Objectives

Upon completion of this chapter, the student will be able to:

1. Review the anatomy and physiology of the heart, with particular emphasis on:
   a. Coronary circulation
   b. Degree of myocardial wall involvement (i.e., transmural and subendocardial)
2. Identify the lead-specific ST elevation parameters

3. Recognize the EKG changes related to an inferior infarction
4. Describe the clinical significance of inferior myocardial infarctions (MIs)

In this chapter, we begin our discussion of the specific types of myocardial infarctions that your patients may experience. In this book's earlier chapters and/or in the companion book, *Understanding EKGs: A Practical Approach*, you learned the essential parameters of basic dysrhythmia interpretation. As we move through this textbook, the picture becomes a bit more complex. We recognize now that critical therapeutic management of acute myocardial infarction depends upon rapid recognition and correct determination of the infarct area. Consequently, the role of the nonphysician intervener as a skilled interpreter of the 12-lead EKG is becoming increasingly significant, because the 12-lead EKG can be used to identify the area of the heart affected by the infarct.

There currently exists an extensive amount of knowledge specific to cardiology including electrocardiology. We would like you to understand that this text focuses on the recognition and interpretation of 12-lead EKGs; we do not presume to include all aspects of 12-lead EKGs in this approach. Rather, we wish to provide you with a practical and workable knowledge of the parameters of basic 12-lead EKG interpretation.

We consciously elected to begin our presentation of the specific types (by location) of myocardial infarctions with the discussion of inferior MIs. In our clinical experience, it appears that inferior MIs are the most common types of infarcts encountered in the emergent setting.

ANATOMY AND PHYSIOLOGY REVIEW

This is a perfect time for you to go back and review Chapters 1 and 2 of this text. You should pay particular attention to the discussion of the coronary circulation. A thorough understanding of the anatomy and physiology of the heart is essential to your comprehension of 12-lead EKG interpretation.

Recall now that the heart is perfused with oxygenated blood through a process known as *coronary circulation*. This process involves the two main coronary arteries that branch off the aorta. Remember also that the two main coronary arteries are called the **left main coronary artery** and the **right main coronary artery** (see Table 9-1). These vital structures supply the heart muscle, or myocardium, with freshly oxygenated blood (i.e., blood rich with oxygen). Inferior wall infarctions are involved with the right coronary artery. Because of this important association, we will now review the distribution areas of the coronary arteries (see Table 9-2).

To review once again, inferior wall infarctions are associated with the **right** coronary artery.

TABLE 9-1 CORONARY ARTERY DIVISIONS/BRANCHES	
Left Coronary Arteries	Right Coronary Arteries
Left anterior descending	Posterior descending
Marginal	Marginal
Circumflex	

TABLE 9-2 DISTRIBUTION OF BLOOD SUPPLY TO THE MYOCARDIUM	
Left Coronary Arteries	Right Coronary Arteries
Anterior left ventricular wall	Lateral wall of the right ventricle
Lateral wall of the left ventricle	A portion of the electrical conduction system
Posterior wall of the left ventricle	Posterior wall of left ventricle
Left interventricular septal wall	Inferior wall of left ventricle

The right coronary artery extends from the aorta around to the posterior part of the heart. Branches of the right coronary artery furnish blood to the lateral wall of the right ventricle. A branch of the right coronary artery called the *posterior interventricular artery* or *posterior descending artery* lies in the posterior interventricular region and supplies blood to the posterior and inferior part of the heart's left ventricle. The right coronary artery branches also supply oxygen-rich blood to a portion of the electrical conduction system.

TRANSMURAL VERSUS SUBENDOCARDIAL INFARCTIONS

You will recall from our Chapter 7 discussion of acute myocardial infarctions that MIs usually follow the occlusion of a severely narrowed atherosclerotic coronary artery. Many factors may contribute to the occlusion, including atherosclerotic plaques, platelet activation, vasospasms, and the formation of thrombi. The majority of MIs (90%) are the result of the formation of thrombi (blood clots).

Myocardial infarctions may be classified as either transmural or subendocardial. Subendocardial infarctions are commonly referred to as *nontransmural*. Transmural (literally translated "across the wall") infarctions involve the entire thickness of the ventricular wall, extending from the endocardium to the epicardial surface. It has long been accepted that the area of infarct begins in the subendocardium, possibly because this area has the highest myocardial oxygen demand, yet the least supply of blood, at any given time. Once begun, and if not quickly disrupted, the infarction progresses outward in a wavelike motion until involvement of the entire myocardium has occurred.

Subendocardial or nontransmural infarctions involve only a portion of the ventricular wall, most commonly the subendocardial layer closest to the endocardium. For purposes of this discussion, you should recall that the coronary arteries lie on the surface of the heart, at the endocardium. Thus interruption of the supply of oxygen-rich blood will adversely effect the subendocardial (or deeper) layers of the heart more readily than the superficial layers.

Once again, let's consider the Q wave. It is commonly accepted that if the Q wave pattern exhibits no changes in an EKG strip, a subendocardial or nontransmural infarction is suggested. However, if the normal appearance of a Q wave has been significantly altered, a transmural infarction has likely occurred. Figure 9-1 illustrates both a subendocardial infarction and a transmural infarction along with relevant EKG tracings.

LEAD-SPECIFIC ST ELEVATION

As you may recall from our discussion of EKG leads, the leads that record electrical impulses generated from the heart's electrical conduction system actually "view" or "look at" specific areas of damaged myocardium. These leads are called *facing leads*. EKG findings of infarction may occur in a

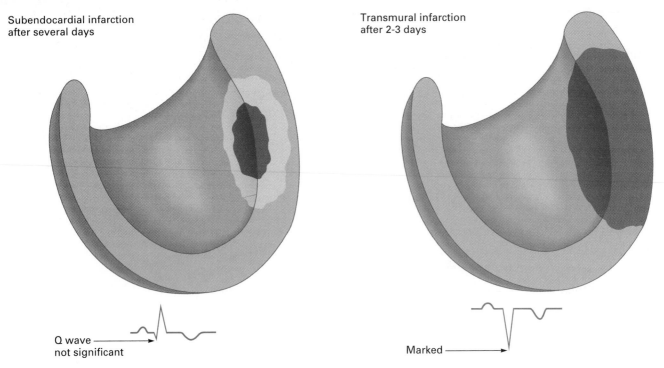

Subendocardial infarction
after several days

Transmural infarction
after 2-3 days

Q wave —→
not significant

Marked —→

Figure 9-1 Subendocardial and transmural infarctions with relevant EKG tracings.

single lead or in a combination of leads; however, for these findings to be significant, evidence should be in two or more contiguous leads. Leads II, III, and aVF visualize the inferior (nearest the diaphragm) surface of the heart.

In addition, Leads II, III, and aVF are anatomically adjacent (or bordering); that is, all three leads view adjoining tissues located in the inferior region of the left ventricle. If ST segment elevation is noted in two leads (i.e., Leads II and V_1) that are not adjacent, your index of suspicion for myocardial infarction will be a bit diminished, because these two leads view different areas of the heart. If ST segment elevation is noted in the lower limb leads (Leads II, III, and aVF), this finding is indicative of inferior myocardial infarction involving the inferior wall of the left ventricle. ST segment elevation is an extremely relevant finding in the recognition of an MI in the initial hours of occurrence.

In simpler terms, if your patient is exhibiting clinical signs and symptoms consistent with a myocardial infarction AND you notice that ST segment elevation is present in Leads II, III, and aVF, your index of suspicion regarding the presence of an inferior MI should begin to increase.

Now it's time for you to look at and study a 12-lead EKG strip that illustrates ST segment elevation (Leads II, III, and aVF) and reciprocal changes (Leads I, aVL, V_2, and V_3). Recall that in Chapter 6 we discussed a systematic approach to EKG interpretation. We advised you then and we'll repeat the advice now: always, always follow the logical and workable 5 + 3 approach in order to correctly interpret 12-lead EKG strips. The first five steps include the systematic approach to basic EKG interpretation. For analysis of a 12-lead EKG strip, we've added three additional steps: ST segment depression, ST segment elevation, and pathologic Q wave.

You will recall that the basic five steps include:

Rate	Rhythm	P wave	PR Interval	QRS complex

The 5 + 3 approach includes:

Rate	Rhythm	P wave	PR Interval	QRS complex

PLUS

ST segment depression	ST segment elevation	Q wave

As you study the strip in Figure 9-2, you should systematically apply the 5 + 3 approach. Now let's apply each of these steps to the strip in Figure 9-2.

Rate:

Rhythm:

P wave:

PR Interval:

QRS complex:

ST segment depression:

ST segment elevation:

Q wave:

We hope you came up with the following answers! If so, you're well on your way!

Rate: 54	Rhythm: regular	P wave: 0.16 sec present; upright	PR Interval: 0.04 sec (4 small boxes)	QRS complex: (1 small box)

PLUS

ST segment depression: Leads I, aVL, V_2, V_3	ST segment elevation: Leads II, III, aVF	Q wave: nonpathologic (within normal limits)

Interpretation: inferior MI, as evidenced by ST segment elevation in Leads II, III, and aVF.

EKG CHANGES RELATED TO INFERIOR INFARCTION

EKG leads that record the electrical impulse formation in uninvolved myocardium directly opposite from the involved myocardium are termed *reciprocal leads*. EKG changes that occur in reciprocal leads are termed *reciprocal changes*. A potential diagnosis of myocardial infarction may be reinforced by the presence of reciprocal changes. Reciprocal changes in the anterior and lateral walls, as noted in Leads I and aVL, may be seen in the event of an inferior infarction.

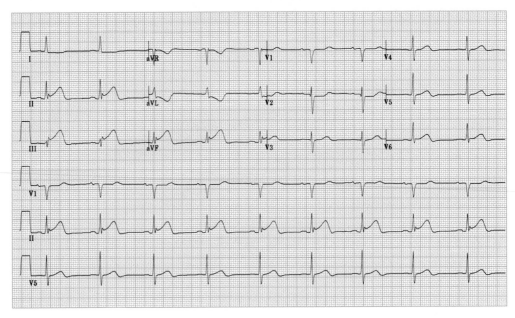

Figure 9-2 Example of 12-lead EKG illustrating EKG changes consistent with inferior MI.

In addition to the occurrence of ST segment elevation, T wave inversion and the evolution of significant Q waves in Leads II, III, and aVF may also indicate inferior myocardial infarction. As a novice student learning the parameters of 12-lead EKG interpretation, it is imperative that you realize the necessity of focusing on lead-specific ST changes.

Although it is important that you look for and recognize pathologic Q waves, you must realize that the appearance of these Q waves indicates that significant muscle damage has already occurred. By the time you see a pathologic Q wave on a 12-lead EKG strip, you should recognize that the MI may have occurred hours previous to this discovery. Nonetheless, in the absence of other findings (e.g., ST segment elevation), the observation of a pathologic Q wave finding must be accompanied by particular attention to the patient's current signs and symptoms, as well as a thorough assessment of the patient's previous medical history.

If the lateral wall is also damaged, EKG changes may be seen in Leads V₅ and V₆. Study Figure 9-3 to visualize the appearance of the EKG waveform changes that may be indicative of inferior infarcts.

CLINICAL SIGNIFICANCE OF INFERIOR MIs

We must remember that our main focus in dealing with 12-lead EKGs in the prehospital and emergent settings is **early recognition and early intervention.** Therefore, EKG findings consistent with ST segment elevation—which is, as you will recall, indicative of ongoing injury—will serve as the hallmark for you to appreciate in order to detect or identify an acute MI in the early hours.

As you have learned while studying this text, early recognition and prompt treatment may prevent the extension of an MI. Your knowledge of EKG changes will enhance your ability to appropriately manage patients who present with chest pain and aberrant EKG patterns.

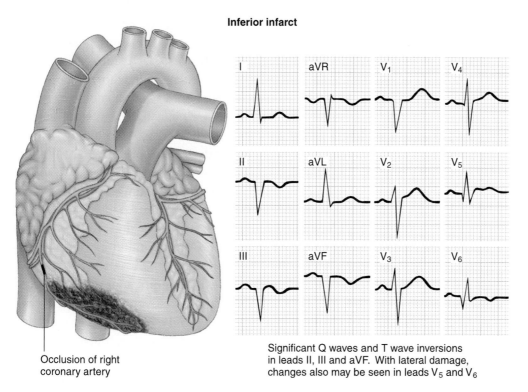

Inferior infarct

I	aVR	V₁	V₄
II	aVL	V₂	V₅
III	aVF	V₃	V₆

Occlusion of right
coronary artery

Significant Q waves and T wave inversions
in leads II, III and aVF. With lateral damage,
changes also may be seen in leads V₅ and V₆

Figure 9-3 Inferior infarct.

Remember always that your patient's clinical picture is the primary focus of your concern. Is your patient clinically stable or unstable? A patient who is clinically stable will generally be alert and oriented and will present vital signs that are within normal limits for that particular patient. He/she may or may not complain of chest pain during your initial encounter. However, the patient who is clinically unstable may present with an altered level of consciousness, moderate to severe chest pain, and blood pressure alterations.

If your patient is hypotensive and is exhibiting EKG changes consistent with an inferior myocardial infarction, you should consider the possibility of **right ventricular infarction** (**RVI**). RVI is a complication that occurs in approximately 40% of inferior MIs and indicates a larger infarction that most likely involves both ventricles. RVI should be suspected in patients who present with changes in Leads II, III, and aVF, because these changes are indicative of an inferior myocardial infarction. Whenever these EKG changes are noted and are accompanied by the presence of hypotension, distended neck veins, and lung sounds that are relatively clear on auscultation, you must have a high index of suspicion that RVI is present.

If you suspect that your patient has developed RVI, an EKG with right-sided chest leads should be obtained. This type of EKG is obtained by simply placing the V leads on the right side of the chest. The V leads most commonly utilized include V₄R and V₅R. This view allows the EKG leads to look directly at the right ventricle and to show ST segment elevation created by the infarct.

If you recall the structure and function of the heart's lower chambers (the ventricles), you may remember that the ventricles function primarily to propel blood through both the pulmonary and systemic circulation. You will realize that any damage to or weakness of the ventricles will compromise the force with which the ventricles contract. Blood flow may thus be interrupted in the ventricles and ultimately compromise perfusion.

When considering the management of the patient who presents with indications of RVI, the health care provider should seek physician intervention for guidance. In an effort to increase preload, the administration of a fluid bolus in conjunction with morphine and/or nitroglycerin may be indicated. Be aware that the administration of nitrates will produce vasodilation, which may produce hypotension. Management of patients with RVI will be dependent upon the treatment preferences of the attending physicians.

Be aware also that RVI may exist without being extensive enough to create significant hemodynamic compromise. This is due to the fact that there are various degrees of severity of RVI. Careful attention to the assessment of your patient is imperative.

As mentioned many times in this text, the significance of early intervention for patients with suspected AMI cannot be overemphasized. Recall yet again that **Time Is Muscle,** and act accordingly. Timely assessment and management, including immediate oxygen administration, must be rapidly initiated and completed within a 10-minute time interval whenever feasible. Your initial assessment and evaluation, whether in the pre-hospital or in-hospital arena, should focus on the **most** important diagnostic tool . . . the patient's general appearance.

A thorough and timely evaluation and management of the patient's ABCs is imperative. Any problem encountered during this evaluation must be managed quickly, followed by a rapid assessment of the vital signs. Because of the wide variations possible in the presenting vital signs, the clinician should be aware that vital signs are not necessarily reliable in diagnosing an AMI. In spite of this fact, it is important that you monitor and record these signs at frequent intervals.

Another very important assessment tool that you will utilize when managing the suspected AMI patient is the cardiac monitor. You must be particularly alert to the presence of EKG changes, as well as to the occurrence of dysrhythmias that originate from ischemic and injured myocardial tissues, because these are common occurrences with acute myocardial infarctions.

Your suspicion of an acute inferior myocardial infarction must be based on a combination of a definitive 12-lead EKG and the patient's clinical appearance, signs, and symptoms. Remember to keep in mind that a negative 12-lead EKG does NOT rule out the presence of an AMI. Remember also that any patient who complains of chest pain must be thoroughly evaluated, and management of the patient should continue until the possibility of AMI is ruled out by the physician.

REVIEW QUESTIONS: CHAPTER 9

1. Two primary structures are responsible for delivering oxygen-rich blood to the myocardium. These structures are the:

   a. Coronary sinuses

   b. Cerebral sinuses

   c. Coronary arteries

   d. Cerebral arteries

2. There are _____ primary coronary arteries.

   a. 6

   b. 3

   c. 4

   d. 2

3. Inferior wall infarctions are associated with the:

   a. Right coronary artery

   b. Left coronary artery

   c. Bundle of His

   d. Coronary sinus

4. Myocardial infarctions may be classified as either transmural or:

   a. Supraendocardial

   b. Subendocardial

   c. Endocardial

   d. Precardial

5. Subendocardial infarctions are commonly referred to as:

   a. Full-thickness

   b. Transmural

   c. Nontransmural

   d. Transdermal

6. Leads that record electrical impulses generated from the heart's electrical conduction system and that "look at" specific areas of damaged myocardium are called:

   a. Reciprocal leads

   b. Facing leads

   c. Viewing leads

   d. Specific leads

7. EKG findings of infarction may occur in a single lead or in a combination of leads.

   a. True

   b. False

8. The most important diagnostic tool that you can utilize when assessing and treating a patient with a suspected inferior MI is the:

   a. 12-lead EKG machine

   b. Cardiac enzymes

    c. Patient's clinical appearance

    d. Patient's presenting vital signs

9. If ST segment elevation is noted in the lower limb leads (Leads II, III and aVF), this finding is indicative of:

    a. Anterior myocardial infarction

    b. Lateral myocardial infarction

    c. Superior myocardial infarction

    d. Inferior myocardial infarction

10. EKG leads that record the electrical impulse formation in uninvolved myocardium directly opposite the involved myocardium are termed:

    a. Facing leads

    b. Viewing leads

    c. Reciprocal leads

    d. Endocardial leads

11. If your patient is hypotensive and is exhibiting EKG changes consistent with an inferior myocardial infarction, you should consider the possibility of:

    a. Right atrial infarction

    b. Left atrial infarction

    c. Right ventricular infarction

    d. Left ventricular infarction

12. Any patient who complains of chest pain must be thoroughly evaluated, and management should continue until the possibility of AMI is ruled out by the physician.

    a. True

    b. False

10

INTERPRETATION OF ANTERIOR MIs

Objectives

Upon completion of this chapter, the student will be able to:

1. Describe the anatomy of the coronary arteries, with special emphasis on the description and distribution of the left coronary artery

2. Identify the lead-specific ST segment elevation relative to anterior myocardial infarctions (MIs), as well as anterolateral and anteroseptal myocardial infarctions

3. Describe other EKG changes commonly associated with anterior MIs, as well as anterolateral and anteroseptal myocardial infarctions

4. Identify the clinical significance of anterior myocardial infarctions

Generally, myocardial infarctions that involve the mass of the left ventricle are considered quite serious. This consideration is based on the fact that the left ventricle of the heart is considered to be the workhorse of the heart—that is, it performs the important function of supplying the entire body with oxygen-rich blood. Consequently, you must be familiar with the indicators that lead you to suspect both inferior and anterior myocardial infarction events. Anterior MIs tend to involve a larger muscle mass than do inferior MIs. In Chapter 9, we discussed inferior MIs; now you will learn about anterior, anteroseptal, and anterolateral MIs.

Anatomy of the Coronary Arteries

Our discussion of anterior MIs will primarily involve **the left coronary artery;** therefore this anatomy review will focus on reviewing the branches of and areas of the heart supplied by the left coronary artery (see Fig. 10-1). As we discussed earlier in Chapter 7, as the left coronary artery leaves the aorta, it immediately divides into the left anterior descending artery (LAD) and the circumflex artery. The anterior descending artery (located immediately to the left of the interventricular septum) is the major branch of the left coronary artery and supplies blood to most of the anterior wall of the left ventricle.

A marginal branch of the left coronary artery supplies blood to the lateral wall of the left ventricle. The circumflex branch of the left coronary artery extends around to the posterior side of the heart and its branches supply blood to much of the posterior wall of the heart. All of these divisions have numerous branches that form a network of smaller arteries and arterioles.

As a reminder, we would like you to look once again at Tables 10-1 and 10-2.

"Widowmaker"

You should remember that the left anterior descending artery (LAD) is the largest of the coronary arteries in the majority of patients. Because of its size and the large amount of myocardium that it supplies, massive infarction of cardiac tissue can result if the LAD becomes totally occluded. Because

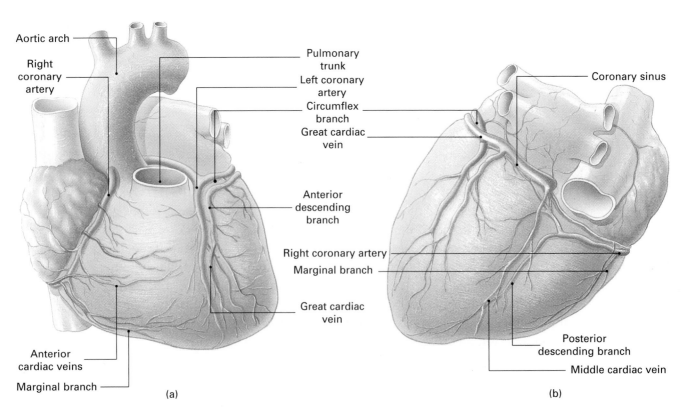

Figure 10-1 Coronary circulation.

TABLE 10-1 CORONARY ARTERY DIVISIONS/BRANCHES	
Left Coronary Arteries	Right Coronary Arteries
Left anterior descending	Posterior descending
Marginal	Marginal
Circumflex	

of the potential for massive infarction, the LAD is sometimes called the *widowmaker,* the implications of which are disturbing and obvious.

LEAD-SPECIFIC ST SEGMENT ELEVATION

As a brief review, the EKG leads that record electrical impulses generated by the heart's electrical conduction system actually "view" or "look at" specific areas of damaged myocardium. These leads are called *indicative* or *facing* leads.

Again, as a reminder, EKG findings of infarction may occur in a single lead or in a combination of leads; however, for these findings to be significant, evidence should be seen in two or more contiguous leads. Leads V_3 and V_4 are the indicative (facing) leads that visualize the anterior wall of the heart's left ventricle (see Fig. 10-2). The reciprocal leads for an anterior MI are Leads II, III, and aVF; however, most often there are no significant reciprocal lead EKG changes with anterior MI.

You should remember that only rarely do MIs involve the anterior wall exclusively. Most often, either the septal or lateral walls of the ventricles are also involved in an acute anterior MI. Leads V_1, V_2, V_3, and V_4 will illustrate ST segment elevation in the face of an anteroseptal MI. This finding often indicates a larger mass of myocardial muscle involvement than does an isolated finding in V_3 and V_4. Leads V_3, V_4, V_5, V_6, I, and aVL will illustrate ST segment elevation in the event of an anterolateral MI. This finding also indicates a larger degree of ventricular wall involvement than does the isolated finding in V_3 and V_4. Both anteroseptal and anterolateral myocardial infarctions will be discussed in more detail in subsequent chapters.

TABLE 10-2 DISTRIBUTION OF BLOOD SUPPLY TO THE MYOCARDIUM	
Left Coronary Arteries	Right Coronary Arteries
Anterior wall of left ventricle	Lateral wall of the right ventricle
Lateral wall of the left ventricle	A portion of the electrical conduction system
Posterior wall of the left ventricle	Posterior wall of left ventricle
Left interventricular septal wall	Inferior wall of left ventricle

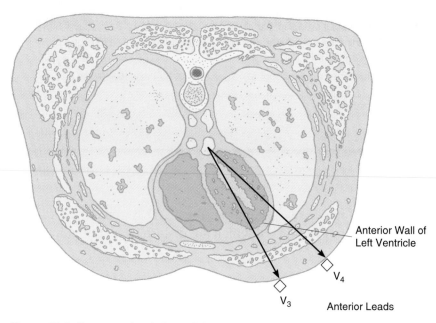

Anterior Wall of
Left Ventricle

V_4

V_3

Anterior Leads

Figure 10-2 Cross-sectional view of the heart with chest leads and associated myocardial wall areas. (Illustration courtesy of Ricaurte Solís, NREMT-P.)

ST segment elevation is an extremely relevant finding in the recognition of an MI in the initial hours of occurrence. In simpler terms, if your patient is exhibiting clinical signs and symptoms consistent with a myocardial infarction AND you notice that ST segment elevation is present in Leads V_3 and V_4, your index of suspicion regarding the presence of an anterior MI should begin to increase.

Let's look at and study a 12-lead EKG strip that illustrates ST segment elevation (Leads V_3 and V_4). Note that there are no reciprocal changes in Leads II, III, and aVF. Again, remember our Chapter 6 discussion regarding the systematic approach to EKG interpretation and remember that you should always follow the logical and workable 5 + 3 approach in order to correctly interpret 12-lead EKG strips. The first five steps include the systematic approach to basic EKG interpretation; for analysis of a 12-lead EKG strip, we've added three additional steps—ST segment depression, ST segment elevation, and pathologic Q wave.

You will recall that the basic five steps include:

Rate	Rhythm	P wave	PR Interval	QRS complex

The 5 + 3 approach:

Rate	Rhythm	P wave	PR Interval	QRS complex

PLUS

ST segment depression	ST segment elevation	Q wave

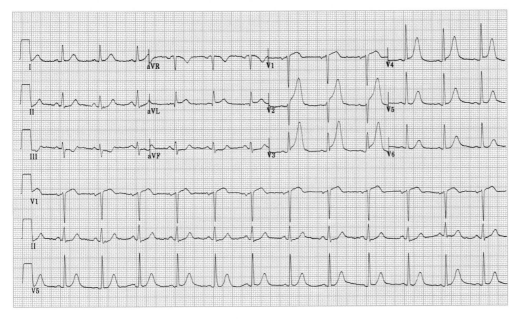

Figure 10-3 Example of 12-lead EKG illustrating EKG changes consistent with anterior MI.

As you study the strip in Figure 10-3, you should systematically apply the 5 + 3 approach.

Now let's apply each of these steps to the following strip.

Rate:

Rhythm:

P wave:

PR Interval:

QRS complex:

ST segment depression:

ST segment elevation:

Q wave:

We hope you came up with the following answers! If so, you're well on your way!

Rate: 74	Rhythm: regular	P wave: present; upright	PR Interval: 0.16 sec (4 small boxes)	QRS complex: 0.04 sec (1 small box)

PLUS

ST segment depression: none	ST segment elevation: Leads V2, V3, V4	Pathologic Q wave: None

Interpretation: anterior MI, as evidenced by ST segment elevation in Leads V_2, V_3, and V_4

EKG Changes Commonly Associated with Anterior MIs

In addition to the occurrence of ST segment elevation, T wave inversion and the evolution of significant Q waves in Leads V_3 and V_4 may indicate anterior myocardial infarction. As a reminder, pathologic Q waves are not an early indicator or EKG finding, but occur as later evidence of myocardial tissue damage.

Another EKG finding indicative of an anterior MI may be absent or poor R wave progression in the V leads. You recall from our discussion of R wave progression in Chapter 5 that the R wave deflection goes from negative in V_1 to positive in V_6, with V_3 and V_4 leads being mostly biphasic (i.e., the R wave is half negative and half positive or in transitions). As the myocardial muscle cells of the anterior wall begin to die, depolarization gradually decreases until the R wave becomes smaller and smaller and the deflection can ultimately be seen as a Q wave. This occurrence is called *loss of R wave progression.*

Clinical Significance of Anterior MIs

Infarctions involving the left ventricle are, as stated earlier, primarily categorized based upon whether the inferior or anterior wall of the heart is predominately affected. (See Fig. 10-4 for a diagram of an anterior infarct.)

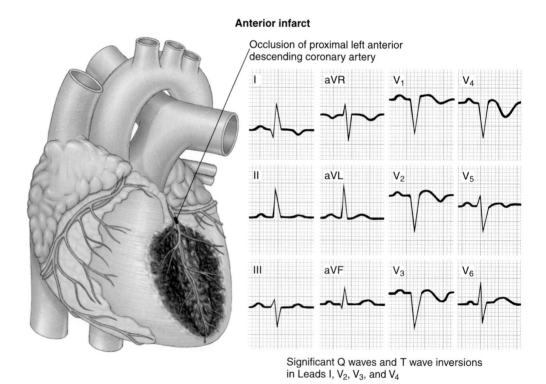

Anterior infarct

Occlusion of proximal left anterior descending coronary artery

I   aVR V_1 V_4

II   aVL V_2 V_5

III   aVF V_3 V_6

Significant Q waves and T wave inversions in Leads I, V_2, V_3, and V_4

Figure 10-4 Anterior infarct.

This is an important clinical distinction because the therapeutic and prognostic implications of these two types of infarctions vary. Because of coronary artery distribution variances, it is a commonly held belief that anterior infarctions tend to be larger than inferior infarctions. Due to this larger degree of myocardial muscle involvement, anterior MIs have a greater predisposition for the development of complications such as lethal ventricular dysrhythmias and cardiogenic shock.

In addition, conduction system defects are more common with anterior infarctions. Generally, first-degree atrioventricular (AV) block and Mobitz Type I second-degree AV block (or Wenckebach block) are more common with inferior infarctions, while Mobitz Type II second-degree AV block, third-degree AV block, and bundle branch blocks are more common with anterior infarctions. As you will recall from the discussions of basic dysrhythmias, both first-degree AV block and Mobitz Type I second-degree AV block (or Wenckebach block) tend to be transient in nature, while Mobitz Type II second-degree AV block and third-degree AV block may need more aggressive treatment, such as artificial pacemaker implantation. Sequential EKGs should be obtained and carefully scrutinized in order to identify indications of a damaged conduction system.

You should be aware that early death can occur in patients with acute anterior MIs due to congestive heart failure (CHF) within a few days of the initial infarct. Also, there is an increased incidence of the development of sustained ventricular tachycardia (V-tach) or ventricular fibrillation (V-fib) up to 1 to 2 weeks post MI. This is an important fact for the health care provider to keep in mind, particularly when dealing with a patient who has experienced recurring chest pain and has returned to the hospital after having been discharged with the diagnosis of anterior MI. Your

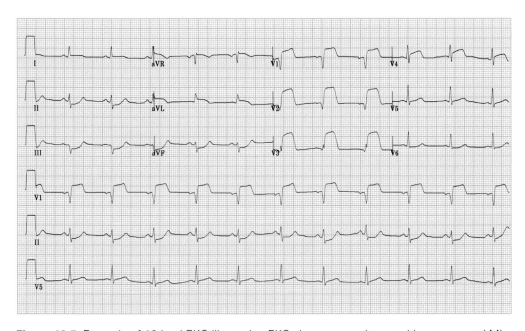

Figure 10-5 Example of 12-lead EKG illustrating EKG changes consistent with anteroseptal MI.

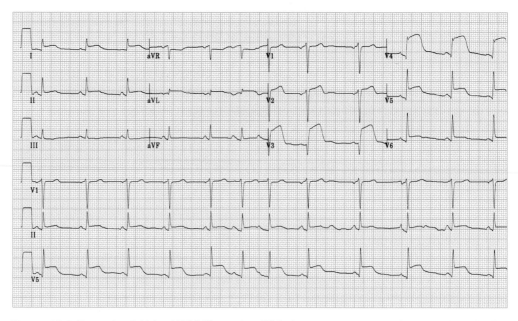

Figure 10-6 Example of 12-lead EKG illustrating EKG changes consistent with anterolateral MI.

index of suspicion regarding the possible development of CHF or lethal dysrhythmias should be increased whenever a patient presents with a medical history of cardiac disease, particularly status post (recent past history of) MI.

You should be aware that the type of autonomic nervous system dysfunction that typically presents clinically in an anterior wall MI results from stimulation of the sympathetic nervous system. Recall that this is the division of the autonomic nervous system that controls the "fight or flight" processes. Thus anterior infarctions tend to lead to hyperactivity of the sympathetic nervous system, resulting in various signs and symptoms including sinus tachycardia and hypertension. Treatment may include medications such as vasodilators or beta blockers.

At this point, you should question yourself as to the significance of sinus tachycardia in the patient who is exhibiting signs and symptoms of an acute MI. Your answer should center around the issue of myocardial oxygen supply and demand. This simple self-test will reemphasize to you the ultimate importance of early intervention and early oxygenation.

You should now utilize the 5 + 3 step approach to evaluate Figures 10-5 and 10-6. Do not hesitate to ask for assistance if you feel unsure about your answer.

SUMMARY

EKG Changes in Anterior MIs

ST segment elevation in Leads V_3 and V_4	T wave inversion; pathologic Q waves may be present

EKG Changes in Anterolateral MIs

ST segment elevation in Leads V_3, V_4, V_5, V_6, I, and aVL	T wave inversion; pathologic Q waves may be present

EKG Changes in Anteroseptal MIs

ST segment elevation in Leads V_1, V_2, V_3, and V_4	T wave inversion; pathologic Q waves may be present

REVIEW QUESTIONS: CHAPTER 10

1. The _____ _____ of the heart is considered to be the "workhorse" of the heart.

    a. Right ventricle

    b. Left ventricle

    c. Left atrium

    d. Right atrium

2. Generally, anterior MIs tend to involve a larger muscle mass than do inferior MIs.

    a. True

    b. False

3. The _____ branch of the left coronary artery supplies blood to the lateral wall of the left ventricle.

    a. Central

    b. Peripheral

    c. Marginal

    d. Secondary

4. The _____ branch of the left coronary artery extends around to the posterior side of the heart and its branches supply blood to much of the posterior wall of the heart.

    a. Marginal

    b. Descending

    c. Ascending

    d. Circumflex

5. Because of its size and the large amount of myocardium that it supplies, massive infarction may result if the _____ becomes totally occluded.

    a. LAD

    b. CAD

c. RAD

   d. MBD

6. Because of the potential for massive infarction if it becomes occluded, the LAD is sometimes called the *widowmaker.*

   a. True

   b. False

7. Leads V_3 and V_4 visualize the _____ wall of the heart's left ventricle.

   a. Medial

   b. Lateral

   c. Anterior

   d. Posterior

8. If your patient is exhibiting clinical signs and symptoms consistent with a myocardial infarction AND you notice that ST segment elevation is present in Leads _____ and _____, your index of suspicion regarding the presence of an anterior MI should begin to increase.

   a. V_2 and aVL

   b. V_1 and aVF

   c. V_3 and V_4

   d. V_5 and V_6

9. Regarding the systematic approach to EKG interpretation, you should always follow the logical and workable _____ _____ in order to correctly interpret 12-lead EKG strips.

   a. six-step approach

   b. 5 + 3 approach

   c. 5 + 2 approach

   d. four-step approach

10. In addition to the occurrence of ST segment elevation, _____ _____ _____ and the evolution of significant Q waves in Leads V_3 and V_4 may indicate anterior myocardial infarction.

    a. T wave elevation

    b. Loss of T wave

    c. Prolonged PR Interval

    d. T wave inversion

11. Due to the large degree of myocardial muscle involvement, _____ MIs have a greater predisposition for the development of complications such as lethal ventricular dysrhythmias and cardiogenic shock.

a. Posterior

b. Anterior

c. Lateral

d. Inferior

12. Anterior infarctions tend to result in hyperactivity of the sympathetic nervous system.

a. True

b. False

11

INTERPRETATION OF SEPTAL MIS

Objectives

Upon completion of this chapter, the student will be able to:

1. Describe the anatomy of the interventricular septum, with special emphasis on the description and distribution of the left coronary artery

2. Identify the lead-specific ST segment elevation relative to septal myocardial infarctions (MIs) as well as anteroseptal myocardial infarctions

3. Describe other EKG changes commonly associated with septal MIs as well as anteroseptal myocardial infarctions

4. Identify the clinical significance of septal myocardial infarctions

Pure (or isolated) septal myocardial infarctions are a less common occurrence than the other types of MIs that we discuss in this text. Generally, an MI that involves the interventricular septum will also involve the left ventricle of the heart. Because there can be 12-lead EKG evidence of a septal infarct, we feel that you should be familiar with the indicators that lead us to suspect both septal and anteroseptal myocardial infarction events. Thus we will briefly discuss septal MIs.

ANATOMY OF THE INTERVENTRICULAR SEPTUM AND THE CORONARY ARTERIES

Our discussion of septal MIs will primarily involve the **left coronary artery** as described in previous chapters. As the left coronary artery leaves the aorta, it immediately divides into the left anterior descending artery (LAD) and the circumflex artery. The anterior descending artery is the major branch of the left coronary artery and supplies blood to most of the left side of the interventricular septum. The LAD also has six branches called **septal perforating arteries.** These perforating arteries supply the anterior two-thirds of the interventricular septum. Still other branches of the LAD are called **diagonal arteries.** These arteries supply blood to the anteriolateral wall of the left ventricle. If occlusion of the LAD occurs high enough in the septum to inhibit circulation to the septal wall, you may note interventricular conduction disturbances. This is true because the main trunk of the right bundle branch and both major fascicles of the left bundle branch lie within the interventricular septum.

As mentioned in earlier chapters, the anatomy of some individuals varies slightly, especially with respect to the distribution areas of the coronary arteries. With this in mind, you should realize that the posterior descending artery, which may be derived from the right coronary artery but is sometimes derived from the left circumflex artery, supplies the superior posterior portion of the interventricular septum.

The heart is generally thought of as a single organ with two halves. The left and right halves of the heart each contain one atrium and one ventricle and are divided by a wall called the *septum*. Technically the heart contains two septa (plural of septum): the interatrial septum, which is located between and divides the two atria, or upper chambers of the heart, and the interventricular septum, which is located between and divides the two ventricles, or lower chambers of the heart. The interventricular septum is larger than the interatrial septum, just as the ventricles are larger than the atria. The interventricular septum has a thicker muscle mass toward the apex or bottom of the heart and a thin membranous part toward the atria. Figure 11-1 provides a view of the anatomy of the heart. You should now refer to this figure to visualize the location of the septum.

Lead-Specific ST Segment Elevation

Recall now that the EKG leads that record electrical impulses generated from the heart's electrical conduction system actually "view" precise areas of damaged myocardium. Remember also that these leads are called *indicative* or *facing* leads.

You should also recall that EKG findings of infarction may occur in a single lead or in a combination of leads; however, for these findings to be significant, evidence should be seen in two or more contiguous leads. Leads V_1 and V_2 visualize the interventricular septum of the heart (see Fig. 11-2). Most often there are no significant reciprocal lead EKG changes with septal MIs.

You should remember that rarely do MIs involve **only** the septum. Most often, either the anterior or lateral walls of the ventricles are also involved in an acute septal MI. Leads V_1, V_2, V_3, and V_4 will illustrate ST segment elevation in the face of an anteroseptal MI. This finding often indicates a larger mass of myocardial muscle involvement than does an isolated finding in V_1 and V_2.

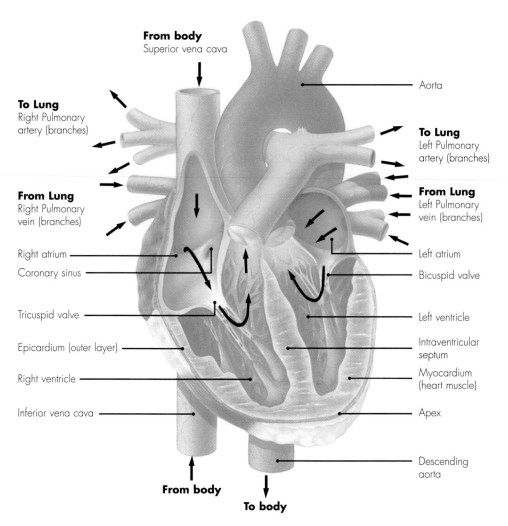

From body
Superior vena cava

Aorta

To Lung
Right Pulmonary
artery (branches)

To Lung
Left Pulmonary
artery (branches)

From Lung
Right Pulmonary
vein (branches)

From Lung
Left Pulmonary
vein (branches)

Right atrium

Left atrium

Coronary sinus

Bicuspid valve

Tricuspid valve

Left ventricle

Epicardium (outer layer)

Intraventricular
septum

Right ventricle

Myocardium
(heart muscle)

Inferior vena cava

Apex

Descending
aorta

From body

To body

Figure 11-1 Anatomical structures of the heart.

Let's look at and study a 12-lead EKG strip that illustrates ST segment elevation (Leads V_1 and V_2). Note that there are no reciprocal changes in Leads II, III, and aVF. As you recall the Chapter 6 discussion regarding the recommended systematic approach to EKG interpretation, you should remember that you must always follow the logical and workable 5 + 3 approach in order to correctly interpret 12-lead EKG strips. The first five steps include the systematic approach to basic EKG interpretation. For analysis of a 12-lead EKG strip, we have suggested the addition of the following three steps: ST segment depression, ST segment elevation, and pathologic Q wave.

You should recall that the basic five steps include:

Rate	Rhythm	P wave	PR Interval	QRS complex

The 5 + 3 approach:

Rate	Rhythm	P wave	PR Interval	QRS complex

PLUS

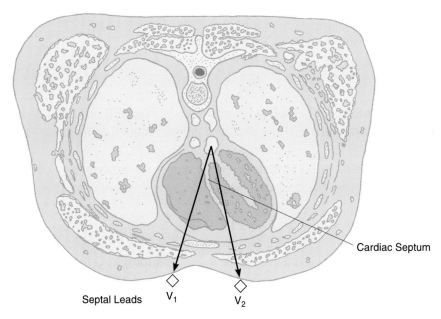

Figure 11-2 Cross-sectional view of the heart with chest leads and associated myocardial wall areas. (Illustration courtesy of Ricaurte Solís, NREMT-P.)

ST segment depression	ST segment elevation	Q wave

As you study the strip in Figure 11-3, you should systematically apply the 5 + 3 approach.

Now let's apply each of these steps to the strip in Figure 11-3.

Rate:

Rhythm:

P wave:

PR Interval:

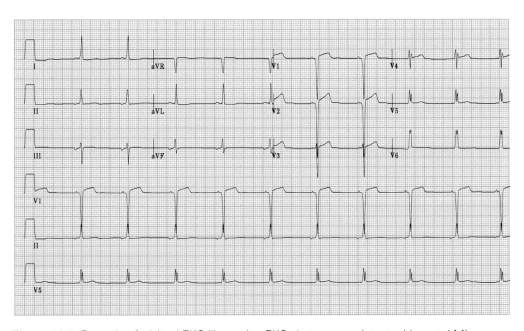

Figure 11-3 Example of 12-lead EKG illustrating EKG changes consistent with septal MI.

QRS complex:

ST segment depression:

ST segment elevation:

Q wave:

Are you comfortable with your answer? We hope that you will agree with the following answers! If so, you're definitely getting there!

Rate: 61	Rhythm: regular	P wave: present; upright	PR Interval: 0.12 sec (3 small boxes)	QRS complex: 0.08 sec (2 small boxes)

PLUS

ST segment depression: none	ST segment elevation: V_1 and V_2	Pathologic Q wave: present in V_1 and V_2

Interpretation: septal MI, as evidenced by ST segment elevation and pathologic Q waves in Leads V_1 and V_2

EKG CHANGES COMMONLY ASSOCIATED WITH SEPTAL MIs

Pure septal MIs, although rare, are recognized by the development of QS complexes in leads V_1 and V_2. Normally, the R wave in V_1 is small yet significant, as it represents the depolarization of the ventricular septum. Another important point to realize is that, while the septum is a thick muscular wall, it is actually a part of the left ventricle. In Lead V_2, the R wave is expected to increase and become more positive (above the isoelectric line). This change or progression demonstrates that the septum is functioning sufficiently well to allow for electrical conduction. This R wave progression is important in your analysis of the V leads. The absence of an R wave in V_2 should increase your index of suspicion for a septal infarction. This concept is referred to as *poor R wave progression.*

In addition to the occurrence of ST segment depression or elevation, T wave inversion and the evolution of significant Q waves in Leads V_1 and V_2 may indicate septal myocardial infarction. As a reminder, pathologic Q waves are not an early indicator or EKG finding, but occur as later evidence of myocardial tissue damage.

As the myocardial muscle cells of the septum wall begin to die, depolarization gradually decreases until the R wave becomes smaller and smaller and the deflection can ultimately be seen as a Q wave. Again, this occurrence is known as *loss of R wave progression.*

CLINICAL SIGNIFICANCE OF SEPTAL MIs

Therapeutic and prognostic implications of septal MIs will be primarily based on the clinical picture of your patient. Due to the location of significant conduction components in the interventricular septum, the predisposition for the development of complications such as conduction system dysrhythmias

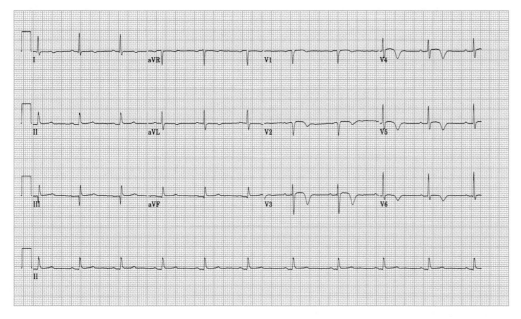

Figure 11-4 Example of 12-lead EKG illustrating EKG changes consistent with anteroseptal MI.

is relatively common with septal infarctions. Generally, Mobitz Type II second-degree atrioventricular (AV) block, third-degree AV block, and bundle branch blocks are the conduction dysrhythmias associated with septal infarctions. As you will recall from the discussions of basic dysrhythmias, Mobitz Type II second-degree AV block and third-degree AV block may need more aggressive treatment, such as artificial pacemaker implantation. Again, your consideration of intervention modalities must be based on your patient's clinical picture.

Recall that pure septal MIs are infrequent; rather, EKG changes will most commonly indicate the involvement of either the anterior or lateral wall in conjunction with septal wall infarctions.

The 12-lead EKG in Figure 11-4 is an example of anteroseptal injury as indicated by ST segment elevation with T wave inversion in Leads V_1, V_2, V_3, and V_4.

SUMMARY

EKG Changes in Septal MIs

ST segment elevation in Leads V_1 and V_2	Poor R wave progression in the V leads

EKG Changes in Anteroseptal MIs

ST segment elevation in Leads V_1, V_2, V_3, and V_4	Poor R wave progression in the V leads

REVIEW QUESTIONS: CHAPTER 11

1. Pure (or isolated) septal myocardial infarctions are a more common occurrence than the other types of MIs.

a. True

b. False

2. Generally, an MI that involves the interventricular septum will also involve the _____ _____ of the heart.

   a. Left ventricle

   b. Right ventricle

   c. Left atrium

   d. Right atrium

3. The left anterior descending artery has six branches called septal _____ arteries.

   a. Penetrating

   b. Protruding

   c. Perforating

   d. Piercing

4. Other branches of the LAD are called _____ arteries and supply blood to the anterolateral wall of the left ventricle.

   a. Perforating

   b. Marginal

   c. Dissecting

   d. Diagonal

5. The left and right halves of the heart each contain one atrium and one ventricle and are divided by a wall called the _____.

   a. Schism

   b. Bridge

   c. Septum

   d. Ridge

6. The _____ septum is located between and divides the two atria, or upper chambers of the heart.

   a. Interatrial

   b. Interarterial

   c. Intraatrial

   d. Intraarterial

7. The _____ septum is located between and divides the two ventricles, or lower chambers of the heart.

   a. Interatrial

   b. Interventricular

   c. Intraventricular

   d. Interarterial

8. Leads _____ and _____ visualize the interventricular septum of the heart.

    a. V_4 and V_6

    b. V_2 and V_3

    c. V_5 and aVF

    d. V_1 and V_2

9. Pathologic Q waves are not an early indicator or EKG finding, but occur as later evidence of myocardial tissue damage.

    a. True

    b. False

10. To diagnose an acute septal MI, evidence of _____ must be present in leads V_1 and V_2.

    a. ST segment depression

    b. ST segment elevation

    c. Pathologic Q waves

    d. Any of the above

11. Pathologic Q waves are indicative of early onset of acute MI.

    a. True

    b. False

12. Electrical conduction system dysrhythmias are a common occurrence in patients with septal MIs.

    a. True

    b. False

12

INTERPRETATION OF LATERAL MIs

Objectives

Upon completion of this chapter, the student will be able to:

1. Describe the anatomy of the left ventricle, with special emphasis on the description and distribution of the left coronary artery

2. Identify the lead-specific ST segment elevation relative to lateral myocardial infarctions (MIs) as well as anterolateral and inferolateral myocardial infarctions

3. Describe other EKG changes commonly associated with lateral MIs, as well as anterolateral myocardial infarctions

4. Identify the clinical significance of lateral myocardial infarctions

Pure (or isolated) lateral myocardial infarctions are uncommon; rather, infarction of the lateral wall of the left ventricle usually involves the anterior, inferior, or posterior wall of the left ventricle. Because there can be 12-lead EKG evidence of a lateral wall infarct, we want you to be familiar with the indicators that lead us to suspect both lateral and anterolateral myocardial infarction events. Thus we will briefly discuss lateral MIs.

ANATOMY OF THE LEFT VENTRICLE AND THE CIRCUMFLEX BRANCH OF THE LEFT CORONARY ARTERY

Our discussion of lateral MIs will primarily involve the **circumflex branch of the left coronary artery.** By way of review, as the left coronary artery leaves the aorta, it immediately divides into the left anterior descending artery (LAD) and the circumflex artery. If occlusion of the circumflex artery occurs, lateral wall infarction will result. The anterior descending artery is the major branch of the left coronary artery and supplies blood to most of the left side of the interventricular septum. Other branches of the LAD are called **diagonal arteries;** these arteries supply blood to the anterolateral wall of the left ventricle.

The anatomy of some individuals varies slightly, especially with respect to the distribution areas of the coronary arteries. With this in mind, you should realize that the posterior descending artery, which may be derived from the right coronary artery but is sometimes derived from the left circumflex artery, supplies the superior posterior portion of the interventricular septum.

In approximately 10% of the general population, the circumflex artery, rather than the right coronary artery, runs along the underside of the heart to form the posterior descending artery. Thus, the lateral wall of the left ventricle is variably supplied by the circumflex artery, the LAD, or a branch of the right coronary artery.

When the lateral wall is involved with proximal occlusion of the LAD, this is termed an *anterolateral MI*. When the lateral wall is involved with a branch of the right coronary artery, this is termed an *inferolateral* (diaphragmatic surface of the heart) or *posterolateral* (superior posterior surface of the heart) *MI*. Myocardial infarctions of the lateral wall of the heart most commonly occur as a result of an extension of anterior and/or inferior wall MIs.

Recall that, of the two ventricles (lower chambers of the heart), the left ventricle is thicker and more muscular. This anatomical variance between the left and right ventricles is appropriate, based on the function of each. The left ventricle of the heart is the "workhorse," and has the responsibility of supplying sufficient blood to perfuse the body. Thus, when the myocardium of the left ventricle is severely compromised, the patient's clinical condition may deteriorate. Note the location of the lateral wall of the heart in Figure 12-1.

Lead-Specific ST Segment Changes

Leads V_5, V_6, I, and aVL visualize the lateral wall of the heart. Although occasionally reciprocal changes may be present in V_1, most often there are no significant reciprocal lead EKG changes with lateral MIs.

Leads V_3, V_4, V_5, and V_6 will illustrate ST segment elevation in the face of an anterolateral MI. This finding often indicates involvement of a larger mass of myocardial muscle than does an isolated finding in Leads V_5, V_6, I, and aVL. Leads II, III, aVF, V_5, and V_6 will illustrate ST segment elevation in the face of an inferolateral MI.

Let's look at and study a 12-lead EKG strip that illustrates ST segment elevation (Leads V_5, V_6, I, and aVL). Note that there are no reciprocal changes in Leads II, III, and aVF. Remember that you should always follow the logical and workable 5 + 3 approach in order to correctly interpret 12-lead EKG strips.

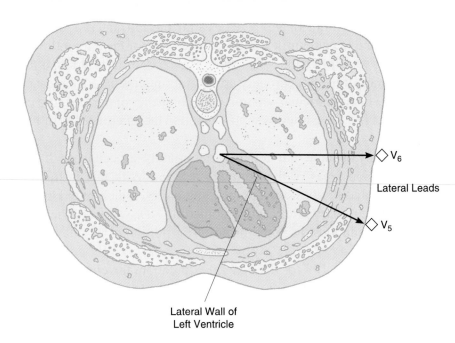

V₆

Lateral Leads

V₅

Lateral Wall of
Left Ventricle

Figure 12-1 Cross-sectional view of the heart with chest leads and associated myocardial wall areas. (Illustration courtesy of Ricaurte Solís, NREMT-P.)

The basic five steps include:

Rate	Rhythm	P wave	PR Interval	QRS complex

The 5 + 3 approach:

Rate	Rhythm	P wave	PR Interval	QRS complex

PLUS

ST segment depression	ST segment elevation	Q wave

As you study the strip in Figure 12-2, you should systematically apply the 5 + 3 approach.

Now let's apply each of these steps to the strip.

Rate:

Rhythm:

P wave:

PR Interval:

QRS complex:

ST segment depression:

ST segment elevation:

Q wave:

Did your answers match the answers listed here? If not, go back and recalculate your findings, remembering to follow the 5 + 3 approach.

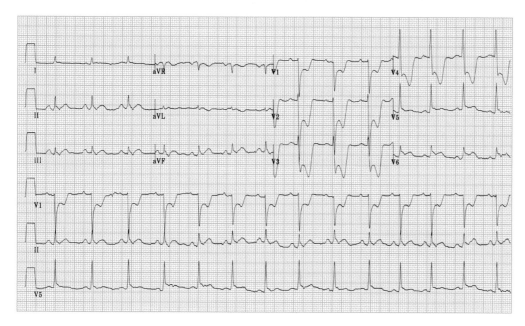

Figure 12-2 Example of 12-lead EKG illustrating EKG changes consistent with lateral MI.

Rate: 83	Rhythm: regular	P wave: present; upright	PR Interval: 0.16 sec (4 small boxes)	QRS complex: 0.08 sec (2 small boxes)

PLUS

ST segment depression: Leads V_1, V_2, V_3, and V_4	ST segment elevation: Leads V_5, V_6, I, and aVL	Q wave: nonpathologic (within normal limits)

Interpretation: lateral MI, as evidenced by ST segment elevation in Leads V_5, V_6, I, and aVL.

EKG CHANGES COMMONLY ASSOCIATED WITH LATERAL MIS

Pure lateral MIs, although rare, are recognized by the development of ST elevation in leads V_5, V_6, I, and aVL. In Lead V_2, the R wave is expected to increase and become more positive (above the isoelectric line). This change or progression demonstrates that the septum is functioning sufficiently well to allow for electrical conduction. R wave progression is important in your analysis of the V leads. The absence of an R wave in V_2 should increase your index of suspicion for a lateral infarction. This concept is referred to as *poor R wave progression.*

In addition to the occurrence of ST segment elevation, T wave inversion and the evolution of significant Q waves in Leads V_5, V_6, I, and aVL may indicate lateral myocardial infarction. As a reminder, pathologic Q waves are not an early indicator or EKG finding, but occur as later evidence of myocardial tissue damage.

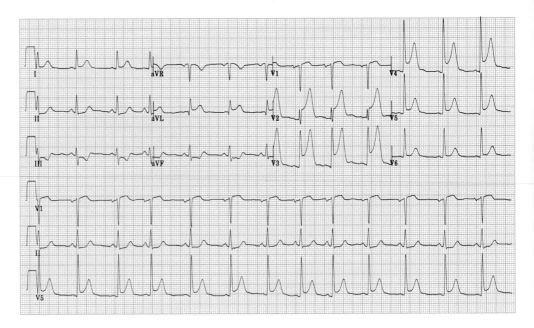

Figure 12-3 Anterolateral MI.

CLINICAL SIGNIFICANCE OF LATERAL MIs

Again, let us remind you that the process of myocardial injury in an acute MI is time dependent. Salvage of myocardial muscle tissue is likely possible if blood flow is restored, but intervention must occur early. Therapeutic and prognostic implications of lateral MIs will primarily be based on the clinical picture of your patient.

Due to the location of significant conduction components in the interventricular septum, the predisposition for the development of complications such as conduction system dysrhythmias is relatively common with lateral infarctions. Generally, Mobitz Type II second-degree atrioventricular (AV)

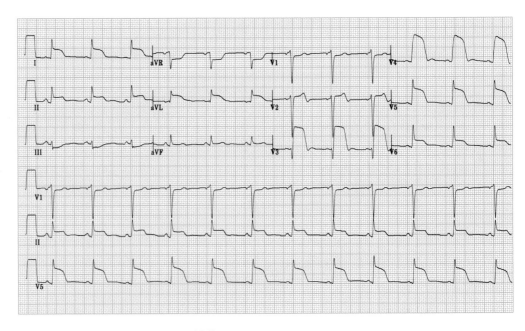

Figure 12-4 Anterior inferior lateral MI.

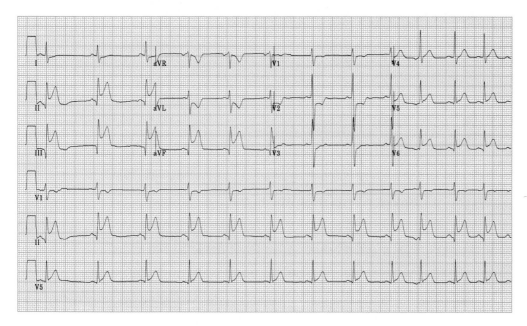

Figure 12-5 Inferior posterior lateral MI.

block, third-degree AV block, and bundle branch blocks are the conduction dysrhythmias associated with lateral infarctions. As you will recall from the discussions of basic dysrhythmias, Mobitz Type II second-degree AV block and third-degree AV block may need more aggressive treatment, such as artificial pacemaker implantation. Again, your consideration of intervention modalities must be based on your patient's clinical picture.

Recall that pure lateral MIs are infrequent; rather, EKG changes will most commonly indicate the involvement of either the anterior or lateral wall, in conjunction with lateral wall infarctions.

The EKG in Figure 12-3 depicts an anterolateral MI. Note the ST segment elevation in Leads V_3, V_4, V_5, V_6, I, and aVL.

The 12-lead EKG in Figure 12-4 is included in this chapter in order to point out to you the significant ST segment elevation that is present, as well as the accompanying ST segment depression. Collectively, these findings manifest the presence of EKG changes indicative of an anterior, inferior, and lateral MI. Note also the "tombstone" appearance of the ST segment elevation in V_3 and V_4. ST segment elevation that resembles the appearance of a tombstone signifies that the occurring ischemia and injury is massive in nature and is a very serious and acute finding.

Another example of a lateral MI, in this case accompanied by EKG changes indicative of inferior and posterior MI, is illustrated in Figure 12-5.

SUMMARY

EKG Changes in Lateral MIs

ST segment elevation in Leads V_5, V_6, I, and aVL	T wave inversion; development of pathologic Q waves

ST segment elevation in Leads V₃, V₄, V₅, V₆, I, and aVL	T wave inversion; development of pathologic Q waves; poor R wave progression

REVIEW QUESTIONS: CHAPTER 12

1. Pure lateral myocardial infarctions are uncommon; infarction of the lateral wall of the left ventricle usually involves the:

   a. Anterior or inferior wall of the right atrium

   b. Inferior and posterior walls of the left atrium

   c. Posterior and superior walls of the left ventricle

   d. Anterior, inferior, and posterior walls of the left ventricle

2. The anatomy of some individuals varies slightly, especially with respect to the distribution areas of the coronary arteries.

   a. True

   b. False

3. Myocardial infarction or myocardial ischemia may be produced by:

   a. Sudden increase in myocardial workload

   b. Spasms of the coronary arteries

   c. Coronary artery occlusion

   d. All of the above

4. Therapeutic and prognostic implications of lateral MIs will be primarily based on the:

   a. Clinical picture of your patient

   b. Serum cardiac enzyme levels

   c. 3-lead EKG tracing

   d. Patient's vital signs

5. Due to the location of significant conduction components in the interventricular septum, the predisposition for the development of complications such as conduction system dysrhythmias is relatively common with lateral infarctions.

   a. True

   b. False

6. ST segment elevation that resembles the appearance of a tombstone signifies that the occurring ischemia and injury is massive in nature and is a very serious and acute finding.

   a. True

   b. False

7. When the lateral wall is involved with proximal occlusion of the LAD, this is termed a(n):

a. Posterolateral MI

b. Anteroseptal MI

c. Anterolateral MI

d. Posteroseptal MI

8. Myocardial infarctions of the lateral wall of the heart most commonly occur as a result of an extension of anterior and/or inferior wall MIs.

   a. True

   b. False

9. Leads _____, _____, _____, and _____ visualize the lateral wall of the heart.

   a. V_1, V_2, II, V_3

   b. V_3, V_4, I, aVF

   c. V_2, V_4, II, aVR

   d. V_5, V_6, I, aVL

10. The interatrial septum is a thick muscular wall; it is actually a part of the left ventricle.

    a. True

    b. False

11. Pure lateral MIs are infrequent; thus, EKG changes will commonly indicate the involvement of either the anterior or lateral wall in conjunction with lateral wall infarctions.

    a. True

    b. False

12. ST segment depression may be indicative of:

    a. Cerebral hypoxia

    b. Myocardial ischemia

    c. Unstable angina

    d. Ventricular atrophy

INTERPRETATION OF POSTERIOR MIs

Objectives

Upon completion of this chapter, the student will be able to:

1. Describe the anatomy of the left ventricle, with special emphasis on the description and distribution of the right coronary artery (RCA)
2. Identify the lead-specific ST segment elevation relative to posterior myocardial infarctions
3. Describe other EKG changes commonly associated with posterior myocardial infarctions
4. Identify the clinical significance of posterior myocardial infarctions

In the previous chapters we have discussed the 12-lead EKG indications that will manifest each specific type of myocardial infarction (MI); however, in the posterior MI there are no facing or indicative leads that are monitored in the standard 12-lead EKG. In other words, there are no leads that "view" or "look at" the posterior wall. Therefore, when considering the possibility of posterior wall MI, you will expect to assess reciprocal leads rather than indicative leads. It is wise to remember that posterior MIs most often do not occur as isolated incidents, but more commonly occur in conjunction with infarction of the lateral and/or inferior wall of the left ventricle. Posterior wall MIs are most commonly associated with inferior wall MIs.

CORONARY ARTERY ANATOMY REVIEW

Now it's time to review once again. Remember that the two main coronary arteries are called the **left main coronary artery** and the **right main coronary artery.** Recall also that these vital structures supply the myocardium with freshly oxygenated blood.

Posterior wall infarctions may involve the right coronary artery, which extends from the aorta around to the posterior part of the heart. Branches of the right coronary artery furnish blood to the lateral wall of the right ventricle. In the vast majority of patients, a branch of the right coronary artery called the *posterior interventricular artery* or the *posterior descending artery* lies in the posterior interventricular region and supplies blood to the posterior and inferior part of the heart's left ventricle. In a small percentage of patients (approximately 10%), the posterior descending artery arises from the circumflex branch of the posterior descending artery.

The right coronary artery branches also supply oxygen-rich blood to a portion of the electrical conduction system. If occlusion of the right coronary artery occurs, the result may be a posterior wall MI, an inferior wall MI, or a posteroinferior MI.

LEAD-SPECIFIC ST SEGMENT CHANGES

As mentioned earlier in this chapter, there are no indicative or facing leads that view the posterior wall of the left ventricle; therefore detection of a posterior wall MI may tend to be a bit confusing to the novice student. We want to be sure that you understand the parameters to evaluate in order to correctly interpret EKG changes that occur in the 12-lead EKG of a patient who is indeed experiencing a posterior wall MI.

Based on your knowledge of cardiac anatomy, you can recall that the anterior portion of the heart muscle lies directly opposite the posterior portion of the muscle mass. Now we ask you to recall that we referred to reciprocal leads as those that "mirror" the facing or indicative leads. Quite literally, what this statement means to you is that since there are no facing leads on the standard 12-lead EKG to detect ST segment elevation and/or Q waves, we must look at the posterior wall's reciprocal leads {V_1, V_2, V_3, and V_4} or modify the 12-lead EKG.

Again, remember that the reciprocal leads are the "mirror image" of the facing or indicative leads; therefore, if the posterior portion of the heart is injured and ST elevation is present, then one could surmise that in the reciprocal leads, the ST segments would appear depressed or directly opposite of their appearance in the facing leads.

THE MIRROR TEST

Although it may not be frequently utilized in the clinical area, one of the oldest and most proven methods utilized to view the posterior MI EKG changes involves the use of a mirror. In order to conduct the mirror test, you should place the mirror above the V leads of the 12-lead EKG tracing and observe the image in the mirror for the presence of ST segment elevation (the opposite finding suspected with a posterior MI). Using the mirror test, you should be able to recognize a posterior infarction by the changes it produces in the anterior leads.

ANOTHER TRICK FOR IDENTIFYING POSTERIOR MIs

Another method of identifying ST segment elevation is to simply hold the 12-lead EKG up to the light, upside down and backwards. In other words, hold the EKG in both hands, with the tracing facing you; then flip the paper over, being sure that the tracing is facing the light. Now look for ST segment elevation in V_1, V_2, V_3, and V_4.

POSTERIOR V LEADS

Another method for interpreting posterior MIs is to actually utilize posterior leads. This method is quite often utilized after the standard 12-lead EKG has been obtained, especially if a posterior MI is suspected. Most commonly, posterior leads V_7, V_8, and V_9 are employed to obtain a posterior view. This is done by taking Leads V_4, V_5, and V_6 and moving them around toward the back or posterior side of the patient's body. This is sometimes referred to as a *15-lead EKG*.

Simply place the patient in the right lateral recumbent position for a brief time in order to apply the posterior leads. To properly place the V_7 lead, you should move the V_4 lead to the posterior axillary position, which is located directly posterior to V_6. For proper placement of V_8, you should move the V_5 lead and place it at the midscapular line. To place V_9 in its proper position, you should move the V_6 lead to the left at the midline of the back, approximately 2 centimeters to the left of the spine.

Figures 13-1, 13-2, and 13-3 show placement of posterior leads.

After the posterior leads are applied, the patient may then be again placed in the supine and resting position. Clinical experience has proven that the patient will rest more quietly and comfortably in the supine position. This position will also tend to maximize the patient's feeling of security and minimize the possibility of muscle tremors, which often lead to artifact.

As with most other procedures in the medical profession, documentation is critically important when utilizing posterior lead placement. The 12-lead EKG machine will not recognize the absence of Leads V_4, V_5, and V_6; nor will the machine recognize the presence of Leads V_7, V_8, and V_9. Therefore you must make marks directly on the 12-lead tracing to indicate that a posterior lead EKG was obtained. *V_4* is marked out and *V_7* is written in its place. The same holds true with *V_5*, which becomes *V_8*, and with *V_6*, which becomes *V_9*. You must understand that a misdiagnosis can occur if a posterior lead EKG is not properly marked. As you have no doubt heard numerous times, **documentation is critical.**

Now it's time to apply the knowledge you have gained in this chapter to the interpretation of an EKG strip that illustrates evidence of both inferior and posterior wall changes.

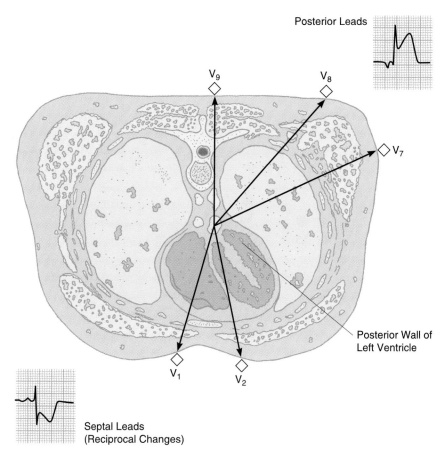

Figure 13-1 Cross-sectional view of the heart with associated chest leads and myocardial wall. (Illustration courtesy of Ricaurte Solís, NREMT-P.)

Always follow the logical and workable 5 + 3 approach in order to correctly interpret 12-lead EKG strips.

Here it is again—just as a reminder!

The 5 + 3 approach:

Rate	Rhythm	P wave	PR Interval	QRS complex

PLUS

ST segment depression	ST segment elevation	Q wave

As you study the strip in Figure 13-4, you should systematically apply the 5 + 3 approach.

Now let's apply each of these steps to the following strip.

Rate:

Rhythm:

P wave:

PR Interval:

QRS complex:

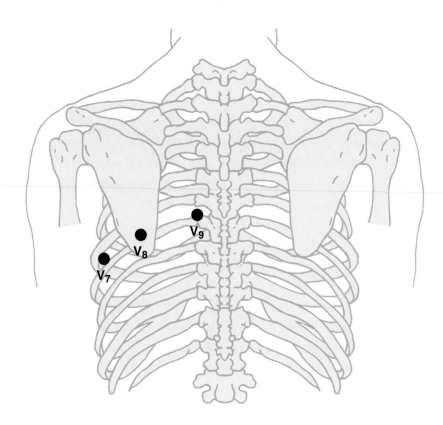

V₇—5th intercostal space, posterior axillary line
V₈—5th intercostal space, midscapular line
V₉—5th intercostal space, 2 cm left of spinal column

Figure 13-2 Posterior V lead placement. (Illustration courtesy of Ricaurte Solís, NREMT-P.)

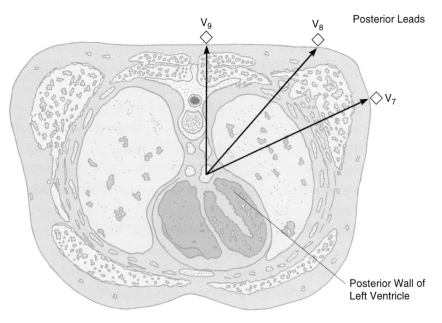

Figure 13-3 Cross-sectional view of the heart with posterior leads and myocardial wall. (Concept and illustration courtesy of Ricaurte Solís, NREMT-P.)

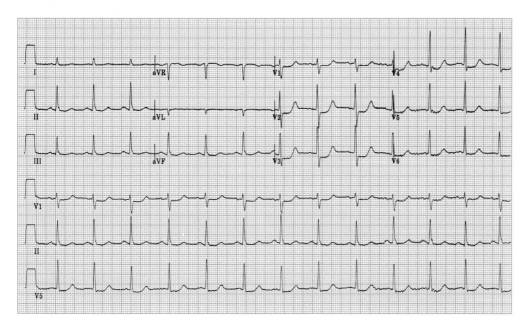

Figure 13-4 12-lead EKG tracing illustrating EKG changes consistent with posterior MI.

ST segment depression:

ST segment elevation:

Q wave:

Now let's see if your answers agree with ours!

Rate: 77	Rhythm: regular	P wave: present; upright	PR Interval: 0.16 sec (4 small boxes)	QRS complex: 0.04 sec (1 small box)

PLUS

ST segment depression: Leads V_1, V_2, V_3, and V_4	ST segment elevation: none present	Q wave: nonpathologic (within normal limits)

Interpretation: pure Posterior MI, as evidenced by ST segment depression.

EKG CHANGES RELATED TO POSTERIOR MIs

As you will recall, in the early stages of a suspected posterior MI (see Fig. 13-5) you would observe for ST segment depression in Leads V_1, V_2, and V_3 (reciprocal leads). Other findings could include the development of tall R waves in the reciprocal leads. When tall R waves are noted in Lead V_1, this finding should prompt you to think of posterior infarction. In the earlier stages of a posterior MI, the presence of tall R waves should be evidenced in conjunction with the presence of ST segment depression. In the latter stages, the tall R wave may be present, but the ST segment depression may have diminished and returned to the baseline.

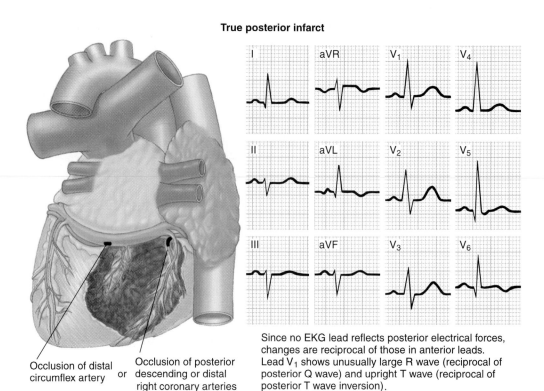

True posterior infarct

Since no EKG lead reflects posterior electrical forces, changes are reciprocal of those in anterior leads. Lead V_1 shows unusually large R wave (reciprocal of posterior Q wave) and upright T wave (reciprocal of posterior T wave inversion).

Occlusion of distal circumflex artery   or   Occlusion of posterior descending or distal right coronary arteries

Figure 13-5 Posterior myocardial infarction.

CLINICAL SIGNIFICANCE OF POSTERIOR MIs

Interpretation of a standard 12-lead EKG obtained from a patient who is suspected of having experienced a posterior MI depends on evidence of ST segment depression in the reciprocal leads (V_1, V_2, V_3, and/or V_4). Various studies have suggested that the placement of posterior chest leads is superior to the use of the standard 12-lead EKG in the recognition of posterior MIs.

The efficacy of prehospital posterior 12-lead EKGs has not been proven. This is true in part because of the difficulty encountered in properly positioning the patient for placement of the posterior leads. However, applying posterior leads in a controlled environment such as an emergency department may be done with relative ease, as described earlier in this chapter.

Again, it is important to remember that pure posterior MIs are rarely encountered. Rather, in most circumstances, EKG evidence will include the presence of either a lateral or inferior MI. You must understand that the clinical significance of posterior wall injury, in combination with evidence of inferior infarction, lies in the fact that this association indicates a more extensive infarction; consequently, a greater risk of complications should be anticipated.

When considering the clinical symptomology of posterior wall infarctions, you should recall that the major area involved in these events is the left ventricle. Based on your knowledge of the anatomy and physiology of the left ventricle, you may reason that necrosis of portions of the left ventricular wall may lead to the development of serious rhythm disturbances that are indicative of ventricular irritability (e.g., ventricular tachycardia, ventricular fibrillation, premature ventricular contractions) as well as left ventricular heart failure.

If the inferior surface of the myocardium has become involved, the patient may complain of "indigestion." This occurs due to the proximity of the inferior aspect of the myocardium to the diaphragm. It is because of the sensation of indigestion that many patients tend to deny the possibility that they are truly experiencing an MI. Rather, they will often self-medicate with antacids. There is clearly no way to know how many patients have succumbed to acute MIs by virtue of this denial. Ongoing efforts toward public education may tend to negate this behavior; however, this may be a rather optimistic point of view!

It is wise to keep in mind that when dealing with inferior, posterior, and inferoposterior MIs, high-degree atrioventricular (AV) blocks (third-degree and second-degree Type II) may be present on admission to the hospital or in a short period after admission. This is true because the AV node receives its blood supply from the right coronary artery; consequently, if the right coronary artery becomes occluded, blood flow to the AV node may be impeded.

In Figure 13-6, you should note the presence of ST segment depression in V_1, V_2, V_3, and V_4. Also, you should note the ST segment elevation in Leads I, II, and aVF. Then you should flip the EKG over, hold it up to the light, and note the ST segment elevation in V_1, V_2, V_3, and V_4. It may be more comfortable (or easier) for you to simply copy the page containing Figure 13-6 and then hold the copied page up to the light.

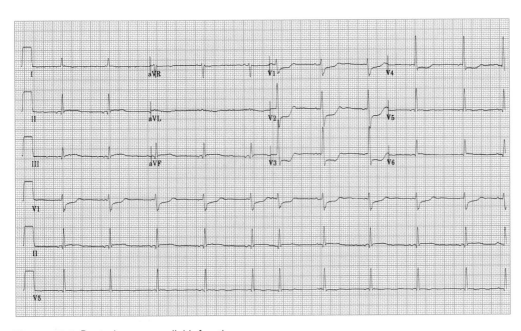

Figure 13-6 Posterior myocardial infarction.

EKG Changes in Posterior MIs

ST segment depression in Leads V_1, V_2, V_3, and/or V_4	Tall R waves

EKG Changes in Inferoposterior MIs

ST segment elevation in Leads II, III, and aVF; ST segment depression in Leads V_1, V_2, V_3, and/or V_4	T wave inversion; tall R waves; pathologic Q waves

SUMMARY OF RECOGNITION OF SPECIFIC MIs

Because the discussion of the specific types of MIs ends with this chapter, there are two more items that we want to share with you. First, look at Figure 13-7 and note the correlation of the chest leads, right-sided leads, and posterior leads with the anatomy of the heart. This figure illustrates the comprehensive views that are possible with 12- or 15-lead EKG tracings. You may recall that, much earlier in this book, we used the analogy of taking photographs of the heart while walking around a pedestal. Think of that action as you view Figure 13-7. We believe that by doing this little mental exercise you will be able to recognize the various views that can be obtained with a 12-lead EKG tracing.

Another aid to memory was formulated by one of our recent EMT-Intermediate graduates, Melissa Patterson. Melissa was struggling to recall the acute lead-specific injury pattern, so she came up with this neat little mnemonic:

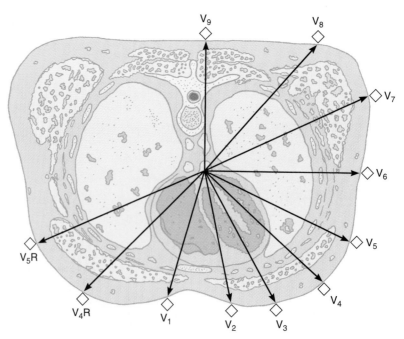

Figure 13-7 Cross-sectional view of the heart with associated chest leads, right-sided leads, posterior leads, and myocardial wall. (Illustration courtesy of Ricaurte Solís, NREMT-P.)

"I SAW A LION'S PAW," or:

I	Inferior	Leads II, III, and aVF
Saw	Septal	Leads V_1 and V_2
A	Anterior	Leads V_3 and V_4
Lion's	Lateral	Leads V_5 and V_6
Paw	Posterior	Leads V_1, V_2, V_3, and/or V_4 (ST depression)

Melissa's classmates (and instructor) immediately picked up on this little mnemonic, and we decided to include it here for your reference.

REVIEW QUESTIONS: CHAPTER 13

1. ST segment elevation may indicate:
   a. Ventricular atrophy
   b. Ventricular hypertrophy
   c. Myocardial injury
   d. Atrial aneurysm

2. The T wave on the EKG strip represents:
   a. Rest period
   b. Bundle of His
   c. Atrial contraction
   d. Ventricular contraction

3. When interpreting dysrhythmias, you should remember that the most important key is the:
   a. PR Interval
   b. Rate and rhythm
   c. Presence of dysrhythmias
   d. Patient's clinical appearance

4. If ST segment elevation is noted in the lower limb leads (Leads II, III, and aVF), this finding is indicative of:
   a. Anterior myocardial infarction
   b. Lateral myocardial infarction
   c. Superior myocardial infarction
   d. Inferior myocardial infarction

5. EKG leads that record the electrical impulse formation in uninvolved myocardium directly opposite from the involved myocardium are termed:
   a. Facing leads
   b. Viewing leads

c. Reciprocal leads

d. Endocardial leads

6. If your patient is hypotensive and is exhibiting EKG changes consistent with an inferior myocardial infarction, you should consider the possibility of:

a. Right atrial infarction

b. Left atrial infarction

c. Right ventricular infarction

d. Left ventricular infarction

7. The combination of posterior wall injury evidence, in addition to evidence of _____ _____, indicates a more extensive infarction and a greater risk of complications.

a. Anterior wall ischemia

b. Inferior infarction

c. T wave inversion

d. Prolonged PR Interval

8. When dealing with inferior and inferoposterior MIs, the appearance of high-degree AV blocks may be present upon admission to the hospital. Examples of high-degree blocks include:

a. First-degree block

b. Second-degree Type I block

c. Third-degree block

d. Wenckebach (Mobitz I) block

9. The 12-lead EKG machine is capable of recognizing the posterior V leads (V_7, V_8, and V_9).

a. True

b. False

10. Placement of posterior lead V_7 is at the level of the:

a. 7th intercostal space, anterior axilla

b. 5th intercostal space, midscapula

c. 5th intercostal space, posterior axilla

d. 3rd intercostal space, midaxilla

11. Placement of posterior lead V_8 is at the level of the:

a. 7th intercostal space, anterior axilla

b. 5th intercostal space, midscapula

c. 5th intercostal space, posterior axilla

d. 3rd intercostal space, midaxilla

12. Placement of posterior lead V_9 is at the level of the:
    a. 7th intercostal space, anterior axilla
    b. 5th intercostal space, 2 cm left of the spine
    c. 5th intercostal space, posterior axilla
    d. 3rd intercostal space, 4 cm lateral to the spine

AXIS DEVIATION AND BUNDLE BRANCH BLOCKS

Objectives

Upon completion of this chapter, the student will be able to:

1. Define the following terms:
   a. Vector
   b. Normal axis
   c. Right axis deviation
   d. Left axis deviation
2. Identify the causes of right axis deviation
3. Determine the causes of left axis deviation
4. Explain the methodology utilized to determine axis deviation
5. Recall and describe the components of the electrical conduction system of the heart

6. Identify the characteristics of a right bundle branch block (RBBB)
7. Identify the characteristics of a left bundle branch block (LBBB)
8. List causes of bundle branch blocks
9. Identify the locations of myocardial infarctions (MIs) that may result in new-onset right and left bundle branch blocks
10. Discuss the clinical significance of bundle branch blocks

A brief discussion of axis deviation is included in this text because this determinant is specific to the 12-lead EKG. Axis deviation cannot be determined with a standard 3-lead EKG. The concept of axis deviation can be very complex. In this text, however, we have elected to employ a simple approach to the basics of axis determination.

EKG Leads

Recall now that an EKG machine records the electrical activity of the heart as this activity is detected by various leads attached to the body. In order to detect this electrical activity, a minimum of two electrodes must be utilized. Thus each lead is made up of a pair of electrodes. Most commonly, one electrode is positive and the other is negative. When an electrical current moves toward the positive electrode, a positive deflection will appear on the recorder. This positive deflection will cause the stylus to move in an upward direction. Conversely, if the electrical current moves away from the positive electrode, this will cause a negative deflection on the EKG machine and thus the stylus will move downward. You should realize that electrical activity of the heart is a complex combination of both positive and negative current flows. These current flows are depicted graphically on EKG paper as it moves through the EKG machine.

Earlier in this text we discussed EKG leads. As you will recall, it takes both a negative and a positive lead to be able to create waveforms on an EKG tracing. Recall also that there are three types of EKG leads. Let's review these now by looking at Table 14-1.

You should remember that the bipolar limb leads and the augmented limb leads (Leads I, II, III, aVR, aVL, and aVF) together comprise the **frontal plane leads** and that these leads are placed on the patient's extremities. Frontal plane leads, as their name suggests, record the electrical activity of the heart in the frontal plane of the body. This means that the electrical currents are measured from the top of the heart to the bottom of the heart, or from right to left.

Also recall that the remaining type of EKG leads, the precordial leads (also referred to as chest leads) are V_1, V_2, V_3, V_4, V_5, and V_6 and that they view the heart in the horizontal plane. In order to envision the horizontal plane, imagine that a cross section of the body is taken from front to back. Now envision the heart as the central point of the cross section. The electrical current flows from that central point out to each of the V leads. A ground lead is used as a reference point or negative pole.

Figure 14-1 provides a view of 12-lead EKG perspectives.

THE HEXAXIAL REFERENCE SYSTEM

As you recall, the limb leads view the frontal plane. The hexaxial reference system takes Leads I, II, and III and Leads aVR, aVL, and aVF and superimposes them over each other to form a 360-degree circle. It is divided into positive and negative sides, with the direction of the left arm beginning at zero (0) degrees. It continues clockwise in 30-degree increments until it reaches 180 degrees, and then it begins to measure in the negative range until it returns to zero (0) degrees. At this time, you should examine the

TABLE 14-1 EKG LEADS	
Bipolar limb leads	I, II, and III
Augmented limb leads	aVR, aVL, and aVF
Precordial leads	V_1, V_2, V_3, V_4, V_5, and V_6

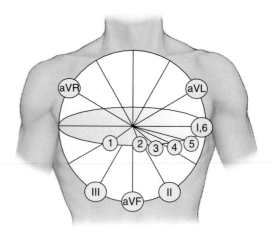

Figure 14-1 12-lead EKG perspectives.

hexaxial reference system as depicted in Figure 14-2 and begin to become acquainted with the leads and their corresponding degree representations.

These degree representations are used to calculate the exact axis of the heart. However, in the emergent situation, finding the exact degree of axis is less important than determining the presence of any deviation in the axis. Therefore, we will now discuss axis deviation.

AXIS DEVIATION

First let's define some of the critical elements involved in axis determination.

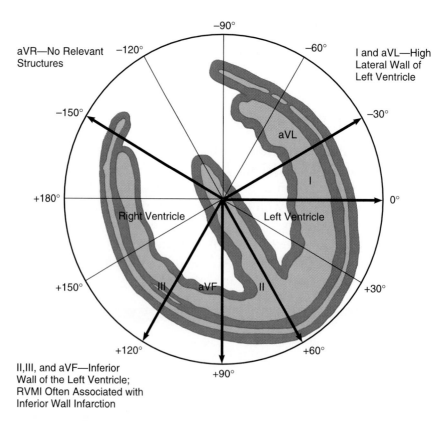

Figure 14-2 Detailed hexaxial reference system. (Illustration courtesy of Ricaurte Solís, NREMT-P.)

Vector   a mark (or symbol) that can be used to describe any force having both magnitude and direction; the direction of electrical currents in cardiac cells that are generated by depolarization and repolarization of the atria and ventricles, as the currents spread from the endocardium outward to the epicardium. Most frequently, arrows are used for this purpose (see Fig. 14-3). The mean QRS vector is typically represented by a single large arrow.

Lead axis   the axis of a given lead.

Axis   the direction of the heart's electrical current from negative to positive.

Mean QRS axis   the mean (average) of all ventricular vectors is a single large vector with a mean QRS axis, usually pointing to the left and downward. As you look at Figure 14-4, you will see the graphic depiction of the normal, or *mean*, QRS axis, which falls between 0 degrees and +90 degrees.

Axis deviation   an alteration in the normal flow of current that represents an abnormal ventricular depolarization pathway and may signify death or disease of the myocardium.

All waveforms have their own axes (i.e., the P axis, the QRS axis, and the T axis). Since the QRS axis is usually the largest of the axes and the most commonly measured, and because of the amount of myocardial muscle, it is called the *QRS mean axis* (which is the sum direction of electrical flow through the heart as a whole).

There exists a correlation between axis (vector) and the anatomy of the myocardium. Recall now that during normal conduction the impulse travels from top to bottom (or from right to left). In the hexaxial reference chart, the mean axis most commonly flows to a point of +30 degrees, which is located between Lead I and Lead II. When the heart is enlarged (ventricular hypertrophy), or due to disease or death of the muscle, the conduction pattern is altered or deviated; hence the term *axis deviation*.

Referring back to the hexaxial reference system, you should remember that the normal QRS axis falls between 0 degrees and +90 degrees. When a change (or shift) occurs, the flow of the electrical current is changed or devi-

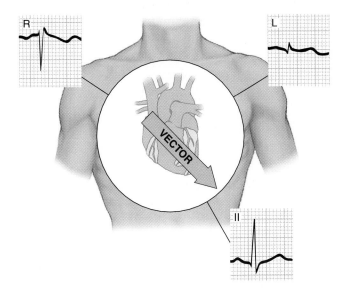

Figure 14-3 Cardiac vector (QRS axis).

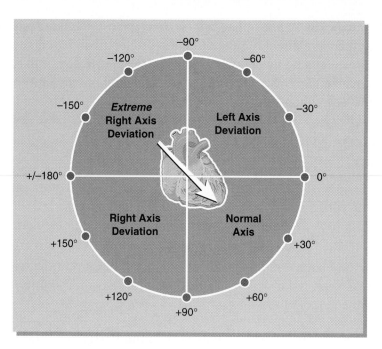

Figure 14-4 Mean QRS Axis.

ated. When the deviation is between +90 degrees and + or −180 degrees, it is considered a **right axis deviation.** Right axis deviation is caused by several cardiac and/or pulmonary disorders. When the axis is deviated between −90 and + or −180 degrees, it is considered **extreme right (or indeterminate) axis deviation.** This degree of deviation, however, is very rare. When the deviation is between 0 and −90 degrees, this is considered a **left axis deviation.** Left axis deviation is caused by several cardiac disorders.

Table 14-2 represents a list of pathophysiological disorders that can cause axis deviation.

There are several methods commonly utilized in the determination of the presence of axis deviation. One method utilizes only two leads, whereas the other methods may utilize more than two leads. We feel that in the emergent setting, the two-lead method is more efficient. Now, let's discuss the two-lead method. In the two-lead method utilized to determine axis deviation, you should look at Leads I and aVF as recorded on the 12-lead EKG machine. Table 14-3 and Figure 14-5 illustrate the findings that may be utilized to quickly calculate the QRS axis.

Determination of axis is useful in 12-lead EKG interpretation in that bundle branch blocks, chamber enlargement, and various other factors can affect the QRS axis.

BUNDLE BRANCH BLOCKS

Review of the Electrical Conduction System

Recall now that the electrical conduction system of the heart includes the following components: the sinoatrial (SA) node, the internodal pathways, the atrioventricular (AV) node, the AV junction, the bundle of His, the right

TABLE 14-2 CAUSES OF AXIS DEVIATION

Right Axis Deviation May Be Caused By:	Left Axis Deviation May Be Caused By:
COPD	Ischemic heart disease
Pulmonary embolism	Systemic hypertension
Congenital heart disease	Aortic stenosis
Pulmonary hypertension	Disorders of the left ventricle
Cor pulmonale	Aortic valvular disease
	Wolff-Parkinson-White syndrome

and left bundle branches, and the Purkinje network. Take a moment and refer to Table 14-4 for a brief, yet concise review of the electrical conduction system, including the inherent firing rates of each of the three pacemakers. Figure 14-6 provides a visual overview of the cardiac conduction system.

Bundle Branches

The right bundle branch runs down the right side of the interventricular septum and terminates at the papillary muscles in the right ventricle. This bundle branch functions to carry electrical impulses to the right ventricle.

Shorter than the right bundle branch, the left bundle branch divides into pathways that spread from the left side of the interventricular septum and throughout the left ventricle. The two main divisions of the left bundle branch are called **fascicles.** The anterior fascicle carries electrical impulses to the anterior wall of the left ventricle, and the posterior fascicle spreads the impulses to the posterior ventricular wall.

Normally, the impulse travels simultaneously through the right bundle branch and the left bundle branch, causing depolarization of the interventricular septum and then depolarization of the right and left ventricular muscles. Simply stated, bundle branch blocks represent the abnormal conduction of an electrical impulse through either the right or left bundle branch. There-

TABLE 14-3 TWO-LEAD METHOD FOR DETERMINING AXIS DEVIATION

Axis	Lead I	Lead aVF
Normal	Positive QRS deflection	Positive QRS deflection
Left axis	Positive QRS deflection	Negative deflection
Right axis	Negative QRS deflection	Positive QRS deflection
Extreme right axis	Negative QRS deflection	Negative QRS deflection

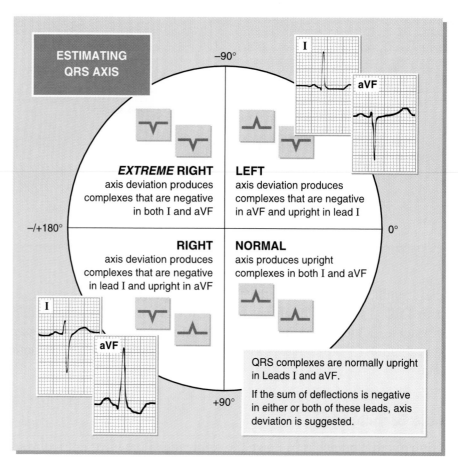

Figure 14-5 Estimating QRS axis.

fore, when one bundle branch is blocked, the electrical impulse will travel through the intact branch and stimulate the ventricle supplied by that branch. The ventricle affected by the blocked or defective bundle branch is activated indirectly by impulses that cross through the interventricular septum from the unaffected branch. There is a delay caused by this alternate route; thus the QRS complex will represent widening beyond the usual time interval of 0.12 second.

Bundle branch blocks may be classified as either **complete** or **incomplete** blocks. While you will not be asked to differentiate between complete and incomplete bundle branch blocks, it is wise for you to know that an incomplete bundle branch block is one in which the width of the QRS com-

TABLE 14-4 REVIEW OF THE ELECTRICAL CONDUCTION SYSTEM OF THE HEART				
SA Node	Internodal Pathways	AV Junction (AV Node and Bundle)	Bundle Branches	Purkinje Network
Firing rate: 60–100 BPM	Transfer impulse from the SA node throughout the atria to the AV junction	Slows impulse; intrinsic firing rate of 40–60 BPM	Two main branches (left and right) transmit impulse to ventricles	Spreads impulse throughout the ventricles; intrinsic firing rate of 20–40 BPM

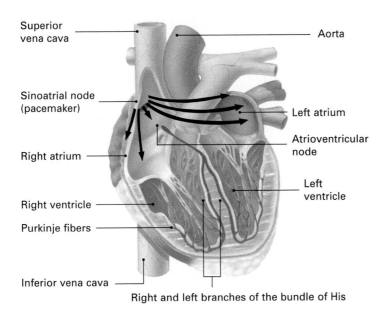

Superior vena cava

Aorta

Sinoatrial node (pacemaker)

Left atrium

Atrioventricular node

Right atrium

Left ventricle

Right ventricle

Purkinje fibers

Inferior vena cava

Right and left branches of the bundle of His

Figure 14-6 The cardiac conduction system.

plex measures between 0.10 and 0.11 second, whereas a complete block is one in which the width of the QRS complex measures 0.12 second or greater.

Right Bundle Branch Block

The occurrence of right bundle branch blocks is a relatively common development. As stated earlier, the right bundle branch leaves the bundle of His and runs down the right side of the interventricular septum to conduct the electrical impulses to the right ventricle. Anatomically, the right bundle branch is relatively thin and is thus vulnerable to disruption. A relatively small lesion can disrupt the right bundle branch. This disruption primarily occurs secondary to an anteroseptal myocardial infarction. More rarely, RBBBs can resemble anteroseptal, inferior, or posterior wall MIs, but they generally do not block the EKG changes of MIs. When an RBBB occurs, the electrical impulses are prevented from entering the right ventricle directly, causing a delay in depolarization of the right ventricle.

As you will remember, the right ventricle is a low-pressure chamber that pumps deoxygenated blood to the lungs. The muscle mass of the right ventricle is smaller than that of the left ventricle. In the normal EKG, the electrical forces of the right ventricle are overshadowed by the more massive forces of the larger left ventricle. In the case of a right bundle branch block, right ventricular depolarization occurs after left ventricular depolarization. In this scenario, the impulse is spread from the left ventricle to the right ventricle rather than being stimulated by the right bundle branch.

EKG changes will occur secondary to the disruption of conduction of the electrical impulses through the right bundle branch.

You may expect to see the following EKG changes in conjunction with right bundle branch blocks:

- Duration of QRS complex 0.12 second or greater (complete block)

- Duration of QRS complex 0.10 or 0.11 second (incomplete block)
- QRS axis normal or deviated to the right
- Small Q waves with normal configuration in Leads I, aVL, V_5, and V_6
- Small R waves in V_1 and V_2
- Classic rSR pattern (see Fig. 14-7) or "M" or "rabbit ears" in Leads V_1 and V_2
- Slurred S waves in Leads I, aVL, V_5, and V_6, producing qRS pattern in V_5 and V_6

Left Bundle Branch Block

The presence of a left bundle branch block may indicate significant myocardial disease. As stated earlier, the left bundle branch is a short, thick, flat left common bundle branch and has two main divisions. The divisions of the left bundle branch are referred to as the left anterior and posterior fascicles. The left bundle branch conducts electrical impulses to the left ventricle and the interventricular septum. A widespread lesion is necessary to block the less vulnerable main stem of the left bundle branch. When a left bundle branch block occurs, the left ventricle cannot be depolarized normally.

The electrical impulses are prevented from entering the left ventricle directly because of the disruption of conduction of the electrical impulses through the left bundle branch. Therefore, depolarization must proceed down the right bundle branch and across the interventricular septum from

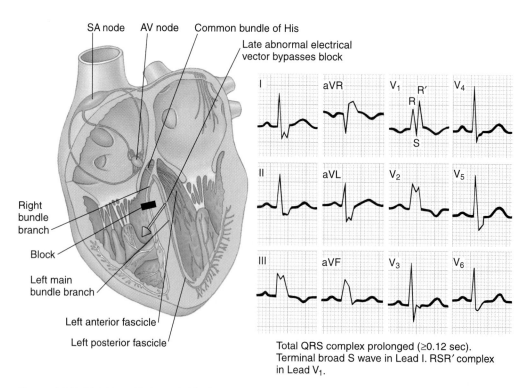

Total QRS complex prolonged (≥0.12 sec). Terminal broad S wave in Lead I. RSR' complex in Lead V_1.

Figure 14-7 Right bundle branch block.

the right to the left ventricle. This abnormal depolarization process via myocardial rather than specialized conduction fibers takes longer, so that QRS complexes are widened and the duration is prolonged.

It will be helpful for you to realize that left bundle branch blocks have the same general orientation as in normal depolarization, traveling from right to left (the same direction as most forces in normal depolarization). Left bundle branch blocks may occur secondary to anteroseptal or inferior MIs.

You may expect to see the following EKG changes in conjunction with left bundle branch blocks:

- Duration of QRS complex 0.12 second or greater (complete block)

- Duration of QRS complex 0.10 or 0.11 second (incomplete block)

- QRS axis normal or deviated to the left

- Q waves absent in Leads I, V_5, and V_6

- R waves small to relatively tall; narrow R waves in V_1–V_3; tall, wide, slurred R waves in Leads I, aVL, V_5, and V_6; R waves may be notched

- Classic rSR pattern (see Fig. 14-8) or "M" or "rabbit ears" in Leads V_1 and V_2

- Deep, wide S waves in Leads V_1–V_3

The underlying heart disease that produces the block, rather than the conduction abnormality itself, usually determines the patient's progress. As a word of caution, you should be aware that the presence of a left bundle branch block will tend to obscure ischemic changes associated with myo-

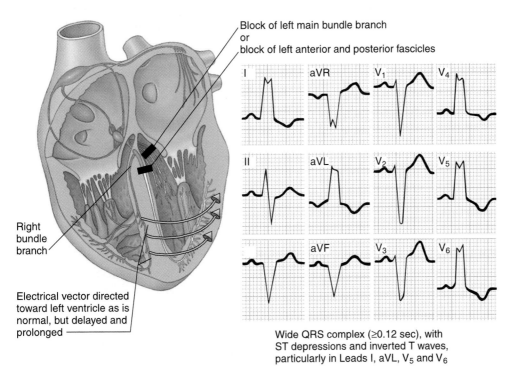

Figure 14-8 Left bundle branch block.

cardial infarction. The possibility of localizing an MI with a 12-lead EKG may be greatly hampered if a left bundle branch block is present. Specifically, LBBBs characteristically mask the Q waves of lateral, inferior, and anteroseptal MIs.

CLINICAL SIGNIFICANCE OF BUNDLE BRANCH BLOCKS

In the prehospital or emergent setting, you should realize that the presence of EKG evidence indicating bundle branch blocks may not be clinically significant. It is very difficult, if not impossible, to definitively recognize a preexisting bundle branch block merely by obtaining a 12-lead EKG.

However, if you encounter a patient who presents with signs and symptoms of coronary ischemia and, after obtaining a 12-lead EKG tracing on the patient, you note evidence of bundle branch block, your index of suspicion for the possibility that this is new-onset bundle branch block should be heightened. Therefore, as a health care provider, you should realize that a new onset of bundle branch block in the face of an acute myocardial infarction is an important finding.

Research indicates that approximately 15% to 30% of patients experiencing MIs in conjunction with new-onset bundle branch blocks may develop complete heart block and an estimated 30% to 70% of these individuals may develop cardiogenic shock. It is also estimated that cardiogenic shock carries an 85% mortality rate. Consequently, you must recognize the clinical significance of new-onset bundle branch blocks, particularly when dealing with patients who exhibit symptomology consistent with acute myocardial infarction.

In order to determine the presence of a new-onset bundle branch block, it is necessary for the physician to have access to previous 12-lead EKGs.

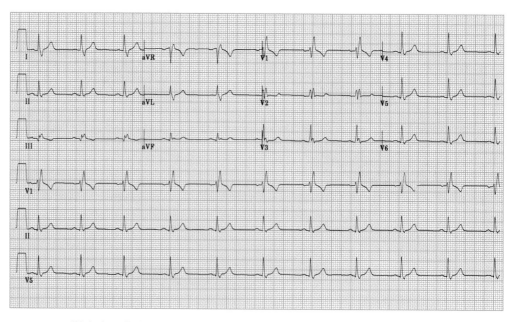

Figure 14-9 Right bundle branch block; normal axis.

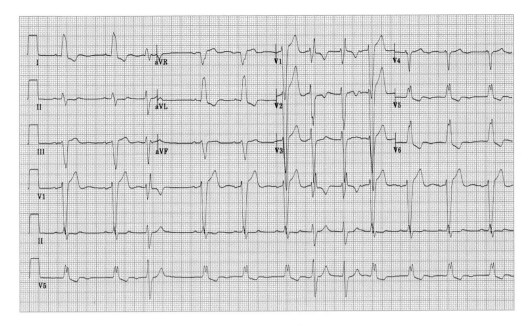

Figure 14-10 Left bundle branch block; left axis deviation.

By viewing a previous 12-lead EKG tracing, the health care provider can determine the existence (or nonexistence) of a previous bundle branch block. Although this is quite important for the purpose of comparative analysis, it may not always be feasible. For instance, the patient may have never had a 12-lead EKG, he/she may be from another state, or the previous 12-lead may be located in his/her physician's office.

The 12-lead EKGs in Figures 14-9, 14-10, 14-11, and 14-12 depict graphic representations of right and left bundle branch blocks.

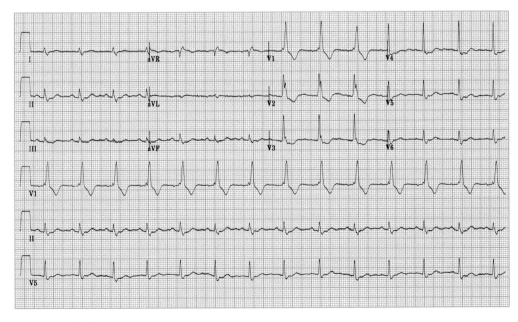

Figure 14-11 Right bundle branch block; normal axis.

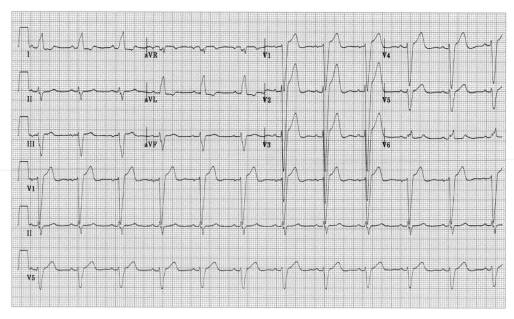

Figure 14-12 Left bundle branch block; left axis deviation.

REVIEW QUESTIONS: CHAPTER 14

1. In the two-lead method of axis determination, a normal axis is determined by:

   a. Negative QRS deflection in Leads I and aVF

   b. Positive QRS deflection in Leads I and aVF

   c. Negative QRS deflection in Lead I and positive QRS deflection in aVF

   d. Negative QRS deflection in Lead I and positive QRS deflection in aVL

2. In the two-lead method of axis determination, a left axis deviation is determined by:

   a. Negative QRS deflection in Leads I and aVF

   b. Positive QRS deflection in Leads I and aVF

   c. Negative QRS deflection in Lead I and positive QRS deflection in aVF

   d. Positive QRS deflection in Lead I and negative QRS deflection in aVF

3. In the two-lead method of axis determination, a right axis deviation is determined by:

   a. Negative QRS deflection in Leads I and aVF

   b. Positive QRS deflection in Leads I and aVF

   c. Negative QRS deflection in Lead I and positive QRS deflection in aVF

   d. Positive QRS deflection in Lead I and negative QRS deflection in aVF

4. In the two-lead method of axis determination, an indeterminate right axis deviation is determined by:

   a. Negative QRS deflection in Leads I and aVF

   b. Positive QRS deflection in Leads I and aVF

   c. Negative QRS deflection in Lead I and positive QRS deflection in aVF

   d. Positive QRS deflection in Lead I and negative QRS deflection in aVF

5. Which of the following disease processes can be expected in left axis deviation?

   a. Left bundle branch block

   b. Pulmonary hypertension

   c. Wolff-Parkinson-White syndrome

   d. Pulmonary embolism

6. Which of the following disease processes can be expected in right axis deviation?

   a. Ischemic heart disease

   b. Chronic obstructive pulmonary disease

   c. Right bundle branch block

   d. Systemic hypertension

7. The right bundle branch runs down the right side of the interventricular septum and terminates at the _____ _____ in the right ventricle.

   a. Purkinje network

   b. Papillary muscles

   c. Anterior fascicle

   d. Posterior fascicle

8. In the prehospital or emergent setting, you should realize that the presence of EKG evidence indicating bundle branch blocks is always clinically significant.

   a. True

   b. False

9. An incomplete bundle branch block is one in which the width of the QRS complex measures between 0.10 and 0.11 second.

   a. True

   b. False

10. A complete block is one in which the width of the QRS complex measures 0.12 second or greater.

    a. True

    b. False

11. In the presence of an acute MI, a right bundle branch block will obscure EKG evidence.

    a. True

    b. False

12. To determine right bundle branch block, the primary EKG leads to observe are:

    a. V_1 and V_2

    b. V_5 and V_6

    c. V_2 and V_3

    d. V_2 and V_4

15

THERAPEUTIC MODALITIES

Objectives

Upon completion of this chapter, the student will be able to:

1. Discuss the purpose of thrombolytics in the treatment of myocardial infarction (MI)
2. Describe and list the indications for thrombolytic therapy
3. Describe and list the contraindications for thrombolytic therapy
4. Review the various thrombolytic agents and the correct dosage of each agent
5. Describe the indications for pacing in the emergency situation
6. Discuss the purpose of transcutaneous pacing
7. Define cardioversion and defibrillation
8. Describe the indications for cardioversion
9. Describe the indications for defibrillation
10. Review the techniques for cardioversion and defibrillation

Recall now that the goal of management of the patient with symptomatic chest pain is to attempt to stop the infarction process. This goal can often be accomplished through interventions such as oxygen administration, pain alleviation, and possibly initiation of thrombolytic therapy in order to limit the progression of the infarct. Although thrombolytics were first used in the late 1950s, it was not until the 1980s that they began to be considered the standard in treating acute myocardial infarctions. In this chapter, we will discuss the five agents most commonly used today.

We continue to stress that the core component of assessment and treatment of the patient who presents with chest pain centers on the prompt oxygenation of hypoxic tissue. Treatment initiatives will vary depending upon your patient's specific situation; however, you must focus on continual and thorough assessment until such time as the patient is clinically stable.

You will learn in this chapter that one of the more serious side effects of thrombolytic therapy involves reperfusion dysrhythmias. These reperfusion dysrhythmias may require various interventions such as pharmacologic agents, pacing, cardioversion, and/or defibrillation. Thus, this chapter will also discuss these various modalities.

THROMBOLYTICS

Thrombolytics have changed the focus of the initial management of acute myocardial infarctions in this decade. Stated simply, thrombolytics dissolve blood clots, which continue to be the leading cause of MIs. This process of "clot busting" allows for the occluded artery to be reopened. As a result, reoxygenation of the ischemic or infarcted tissue will likely occur. You have learned in previous chapters the critical importance of the **Time Is Muscle** concept. The maximum benefit of thrombolytic therapy is best achieved when the agent is administered within 6 hours after onset of symptoms. Now we will focus on several of the thrombolytic agents that you will likely be encountering when dealing with the emergent treatment of acute MI.

Indications

The administration of thrombolytics may be indicated, based on specific screening criteria, for the patient who presents with clinical and EKG evidence of an acute myocardial infarction. Clinical presentations in patients with suspected acute MIs were discussed in detail in Chapter 8. Based again on the **Time Is Muscle** concept, you will recognize that late EKG changes (i.e., the development of pathologic Q waves) occur hours after the initial insult. To wait for this type of definitive EKG change would therefore be detrimental to the very purpose of thrombolytic therapy (early interruption of the MI process). Thus the most commonly utilized tool to indicate the presence of myocardial damage that may lead to infarction is ST segment elevation.

Table 15-1 presents some indications for thrombolytic therapy.

Screening Criteria

Screening criteria for the use of thrombolytic therapy are very important and essential components of the selection of potential candidates. The major side effect of thrombolytic therapy is bleeding. These agents not only dissolve clots located in the coronary arteries, but also clots in any circulatory system vessel. Consequently, the screening is done to identify those patients who may be susceptible to catastrophic hemorrhage.

TABLE 15-1 INDICATIONS FOR THROMBOLYTIC THERAPY	
ST segment elevation (1 mm or greater in 2 contiguous leads)	Clinical presentation: chest pain unrelieved by rest (may radiate), diaphoresis, pallor

Thrombolytic check sheets are composed of generic lists of patient data, as well as lists of absolute and relative contraindications. The format of the check sheet may vary. The information inquiry, based on the particular check sheet, is typically completed in the prehospital setting or immediately upon arrival in the critical care areas of the hospital [emergency department (ED), intensive care unit (ICU), constant care unit (CCU)].

Contraindications

Although contraindications are numerous and very notable, it is vital to stress the importance of the proven beneficial role of thrombolytic therapy in the treatment of acute myocardial infarction. The major complication of thrombolytic therapy is hemorrhage—usually a direct result of the mechanism of action of the agent.

Contraindications in the use of thrombolytic therapy are classified as absolute and relative. Relative contraindications are those that the physician must consider in the decision to institute or withhold thrombolytic therapy. With the existence of as few as one of the absolute contraindications, thrombolytic therapy is usually not initiated. As with any type of therapy, however, the physician must ultimately decide whether the benefits of thrombolytic therapy in fact outweigh the risks. If the physician decides that thrombolytic therapy is the treatment modality of choice, he/she must consult the patient regarding this decision and seek to gain permission.

Tables 15-2 and 15-3 depict the most commonly used relative and absolute contraindications.

Thrombolytic Agents

Acetylsalicylic acid (ASA, Aspirin)
Aspirin is one of the most commonly used anti-inflammatory agents. One of the primary mechanisms of action of acetylsalicytic acid is its ability to inhibit the function of platelets. Thus ASA has gained prominence as a beneficial agent in the treatment of thromboembolic diseases such as acute

TABLE 15-2 EXAMPLES OF INCLUSION CRITERIA FOR THROMBOLYTIC THERAPY
Inclusion Criteria
• Age less than 75 years

• Clinical complaints consistent with ischemic-type chest pain
  – Onset of chest pain occurring within 12 hr
  – Most benefit from thrombolysis if given within 6 hr
  – Little benefit from thrombolysis if given after 12 hr, unless symptomatic

• EKG changes
  – ST segment elevation ≥ 1 mm in 2 or more contiguous limb leads
  – ST-segment elevation ≥ 2 mm in 2 or more contiguous precordial leads
  – New or presumably new bundle branch block (BBB)

TABLE 15-3 EXAMPLES OF EXCLUSION CRITERIA FOR THROMBOLYTIC THERAPY

Relative Contraindications	Absolute Contraindications
• Severe uncontrolled hypertension at presentation (BP > 180/110)	• Unwilling or unable to give informed consent
• Other intracerebral pathology	• Previous hemorrhagic stroke at any time; other strokes or cerebrovascular events within 1 yr
• Current use of anticoagulants	• Known intracranial neoplasm
• Recent trauma (2–4 wk), including head trauma	• Active internal bleeding
• Prolonged and traumatic cardiopulmonary resuscitation (CPR)	• Suspected aortic dissection
• Major surgery (<3 wk prior)	
• Noncompressible vascular punctures	
• Recent (2–4 wk) internal bleeding	
• Pregnancy	
• Active peptic ulcer	

myocardial infarction. It has proven highly effective in reducing mortality associated with myocardial infarction. Aspirin also appears to reduce the rate of nonfatal stroke.

TRADE NAME:	Aspirin
GENERIC NAME:	Acetylsalicytic acid
ONSET:	5 to 30 minutes after ingestion
HALF-LIFE:	2 to 3 hours for low dosages
DOSAGE:	325 milligrams (chewable)
SIDE EFFECTS:	Tinnitus, dizziness, gastrointestinal (GI) disorders
PRECAUTIONS:	History of GI disease, renal disease, hepatic disease, chronic alcohol use and abuse

Streptokinase (SK)
Streptokinase (SK) was the first thrombolytic agent on the market and available for use. This agent has a bacterial origin. Anisoylated plasminogen SK activator complex (APSAC) was developed after SK as a hybrid.

TRADE NAME:	Streptase
GENERIC NAME:	Streptokinase
ONSET:	Immediate
PEAK:	20 minutes to 2 hours
DURATION:	4 hours
DOSAGE:	1.5 million units in 1-hour infusion

SIDE EFFECTS: Bleeding, allergic reaction, anaphylaxis, fever, nausea, vomiting

PRECAUTIONS: Streptase therapy within past 12 months; anaphylaxis may occur; reperfusion dysrhythmias are common

Tissue Plasminogen Activator (tPA, Alteplase)

tPA/Alteplase has the distinction of being considered a clot-specific agent at low doses. This means that tPA will work on those clots in the coronary arteries that were recently formed and leave other clots in the systemic circulation alone. However, at therapeutic levels, tPA does not noticeably decrease the incidence of bleeding when compared with either SK or urokinase (UK).

TRADE NAME: Activase

GENERIC NAME: Alteplase, tissue plasminogen activator

ONSET: Immediate

PEAK: 45 minutes

DURATION: 4 hours

DOSAGE: 15-milligram intravenous (IV) bolus over 1 to 2 minutes;

then 0.75 milligrams per kilogram over 30 minutes (not to exceed 50 milligrams);

then 0.5 milligrams per kilogram over 60 minutes (not to exceed 35 milligrams)

SIDE EFFECTS: Bleeding, allergic reaction (infrequent), fever, nausea, vomiting, hypotension

PRECAUTIONS: Although very uncommon, anaphylaxis may occur; reperfusion dysrhythmias are common

Retavase

Retavase, one of the newest agents, was approved by the Food and Drug Administration in the latter part of 1996. This thrombolytic agent is given as a double bolus of 10 units each, with the second bolus given 30 minutes after the first.

TRADE NAME: Retavase

GENERIC NAME: Reteplase, Recombinant

ONSET: Immediate

PEAK: 80 minutes

DURATION: Half-life is 13 to 16 minutes

DOSAGE: 10-unit IV bolus over 1 to 2 minutes;

wait 30 minutes, then repeat dosage (10-unit IV bolus over 1 to 2 minutes)

SIDE EFFECTS: Bleeding, allergic reactions

PRECAUTIONS: Heparin and Retavase are incompatible when combined in solution and should not be administered simultaneously in the same IV line; reperfusion dysrhythmias are common

TNK {TNKase}/TNK-t-PA

TNK-t-PA is the newest thrombolytic agent on the market, released for use in early 2000.

TRADE NAME:	TNKase (TNK-t-PA)
GENERIC NAME:	Tenecteptase
ONSET:	16 minutes
DURATION:	Half-life is 20 minutes
DOSAGE:	0.50 to 0.55 milligrams per kilogram (body weight adjusted) single dose over 5 seconds. Recommended total dose should not exceed 50 mg.
SIDE EFFECTS:	Bleeding, allergic reaction (infrequent), fever, nausea, vomiting, hypotension
PRECAUTIONS:	Reperfusion dysrhythmias

Urokinase (UK)

Although UK has been available for a longer period of time than either tPA or APSAC, this agent has been involved in the least amount of trial testing.

EMERGENCY EXTERNAL CARDIAC PACING

As we noted in the discussion of thrombolytic agents, one of the most common precautions that we must be aware of is the prevalence of reperfusion dysrhythmias, particularly the bradydysrhythmias. Consequently, a discussion of external cardiac pacing is a necessary component of this chapter.

Although the concept of emergency cardiac pacing has been around for more than a century, the use of this therapy has become much more standard in the past decade. Although there are several different types of cardiac pacing, the type used most often in the emergent setting is called transcutaneous cardiac pacing (TCP). Among the more advantageous features of TCP are the minimal occurrence of complications, the procedure's documented effectiveness, and the small amount of time needed to initiate the therapy.

Transcutaneous pacing is performed via two large electrode pads that are most commonly placed in an anterior-posterior position on the patient's chest to conduct electrical impulses through the skin to the heart. When this method is used, cardiac cells depolarize in a normal fashion. Prior to implementation of TCP, the patient should be placed in a supine position and IV, oxygen, and EKG monitoring must be established. It is essential for the health care provider to have received either Medical Control orders or orders from the attending physician prior to initiating TCP.

Indications for External Cardiac Pacing

External cardiac pacing (TCP) is sometimes indicated for the treatment of certain reperfusion dysrhythmias, such as symptomatic bradycardia and/or heart block associated with reduced cardiac output. Examples of bradydysrhythmias frequently seen following the administration of thrombolytics include {but are not limited to}:

- Third-degree (complete) heart block
- Second-degree Mobitz Type II heart block
- Idioventricular rhythm (IVR)
- Accelerated idioventricular rhythm (AIVR)
- Profound bradycardia (clinically symptomatic)

It is important to note that you must carefully observe your patient throughout the initiation of thrombolytic therapy. In the event that reperfusion dysrhythmias occur following the administration of a thrombolytic agent, it is imperative that you immediately identify the rhythm. If the rhythm is a bradydysrhythmia and the patient is exhibiting symptoms of hypoperfusion (alterations in mental status, chest pain, decreasing blood pressure), you must consider treating the patient with TCP either in conjunction with or following drug therapy. As always, you should follow your local protocols and/or medical direction. It is also critical that you assure that your patient is receiving proper and adequate oxygenation.

Table 15-4 displays the procedure for transcutaneous pacing.

TABLE 15-4 PROCEDURE FOR TRANSCUTANEOUS PACING

Step 1: Ensure monitoring electrodes are in place.

Step 2: Attach pacing electrodes (preferred placement is anterior-posterior).*

Step 3: Turn the pacing unit on (method will vary based on type of monitor).

Step 4: Adjust QRS size to allow the monitor to sense the present QRS complex.

Step 5: Set the rate to the desired value (usually 70–80 BPM).

Step 6: Set the milliamps (mA) to 70–80 mA (usual setting).

Step 7: Increase the mA by increments of 5–10 mA (unit dependent) until capture occurs.

Step 8: Assess for capture by observing the characteristically widened QRS complex (see Figure 15-1) and assess for presence of carotid pulse.

Step 9: Keep mA at a minimum (5–10 mA above the level needed for capture).

Step 10: Consider sedation as per medical direction or local protocol.

*The anterior electrode is placed to the left of the sternum at the fifth intercostal space, midclavicular; the posterior electrode is placed on the back, to the left of the spine, below the clavicle and in line with anterior electrode (see Fig. 15-2).

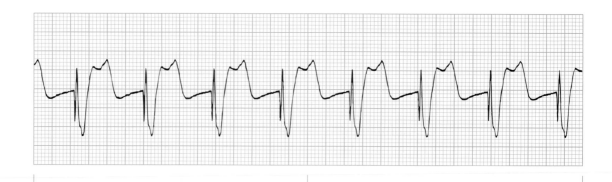

Figure 15-1 Normal capturing pacer rhythm.

Complications of Transcutaneous Pacing

One of the more common complications of transcutaneous pacing is pain. With the delivery of electrical current through the skin into the heart, the patient will experience discomfort secondary to both the electrical stimulus and muscle contractions. It is for this reason that analgesics and/or sedatives are often administered prior to and during TCP. Another potential complication that sometimes occurs is failure to capture (when the pacemaker fails to successfully depolarize the myocardium). The major causes of failure to capture in TCP therapy are poor or incorrect pad placement and patient movement.

DEFIBRILLATION

Defibrillation, also known as *asynchronous cardioversion,* is a therapeutic modality by virtue of its ability to terminate fibrillation by passing a current of electricity through the heart's critical mass. Recall now that ventricular fibrillation is a life-threatening dysrhythmia. When the cells of the heart's critical mass (multiple cells) are discharging independently of other cardiac cells, ventricular fibrillation ensues. Because there is no organization of

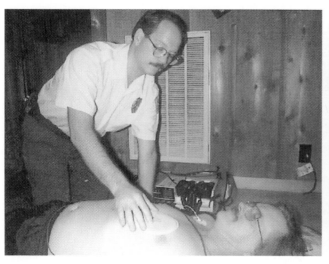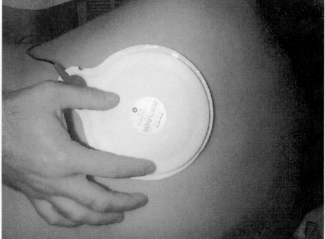

Figure 15-2 Anterior-posterior electrode placement.

depolarization or repolarization leading to myocardial contraction, there can be no significant cardiac output. Subsequently, if your patient's heart is unable to produce any output, your patient's viability will soon diminish and perfusion will cease. Without appropriate treatment (airway, oxygen, defibrillation), asystole will soon follow ventricular fibrillation.

It is widely agreed that the most frequent rhythm associated with sudden cardiac death is ventricular fibrillation. Currently, electrical defibrillation is the most effective method of terminating ventricular fibrillation. Because pulseless ventricular tachycardia (VT, V-tach) rapidly deteriorates into ventricular fibrillation (VF, V-fib), if either of these rhythms are left untreated, asystole will rapidly develop. Therefore, both pulseless VT and VF must be rapidly controlled with defibrillation.

The success of defibrillation is extremely time dependent. Numerous studies have documented the fact that defibrillation is most successful if delivered within the first minute after cardiac arrest has occurred. Unfortunately, after only 8 to 9 minutes of cardiac arrest, a successful resuscitation occurs in less than 1 out of every 10 attempts. While CPR is critically important and necessary in a cardiac arrest situation, you should realize that CPR is most effective in maintaining coronary and cerebral blood flow rather than in actually converting ventricular fibrillation. It is important to stress, therefore, that effective CPR must be implemented and maintained until a defibrillator is available. Early defibrillation is essential.

A variety of defibrillators are available for purchase and use in today's market. These various defibrillators have several energy level settings that the health care provider selects before charging the capacitor and delivering the energy. The specific amount of energy is selected based upon patient needs and is measured in **joules,** or watt-seconds. The common maximum energy level used for defibrillation is 360 watt-seconds.

As you might imagine, the higher the amount of energy selected, the more energy will be delivered to the heart. You must keep in mind that the more electrical energy that is delivered to the myocardium, the greater the risk of myocardial damage. It is for this reason that we elect to begin with an energy level that is likely to convert the rhythm from fibrillation but is not so high that it will cause unnecessary myocardial tissue damage.

For the initial defibrillation attempt in a patient with pulseless VT or VF, 200 joules is used. The second defibrillation attempt should be 200 to 300 joules, and the third and highest energy level is 360 joules. After these three "stacked" shocks have been delivered, successive defibrillations are delivered at 360 joules. *Stacked shocks* refer to three consecutive shocks that are delivered without pausing between each defibrillation. If the VF or pulseless VT recurs following successful conversion, you should select the energy level that was previously successful.

Transthoracic Resistance

As is well known, electricity will travel along the pathway of least resistance. The chest can offer a high resistance to electrical flow (called *transthoracic resistance*) during defibrillation attempts. Energy delivered during defibrillation must pass through the chest wall before it reaches the heart. A portion of the energy delivered is used up in overcoming the high transthoracic resistance of the chest. Thus the amount of current that actually reaches the heart during defibrillation is less than the initial current that was delivered through the paddles. If this resistance to current flow is not lowered during the defibrillation process, a subtherapeutic amount of energy may reach the heart and it may thus be impossible to defibrillate the critical mass of myocardial tissue.

There are many factors that may determine the amount of transthoracic resistance to current flow. Some of these factors are electrode position, electrode size, interface material between the electrode and the skin, size of the patient, contact pressure, successive defibrillations, and energy level selection.

Simply ensuring that the electrode applied to the patient's chest is the proper size can decrease resistance. Electrode paddles for the adult patient should be 8.5 to 12 centimeters in diameter. Infant paddles, which typically clip onto the adult paddle and have a smaller surface area, are typically 4.5 centimeters in diameter, while child-size electrodes have a diameter of about 8 centimeters. Whatever size electrode is used, it is essential that there be no large voids between the chest wall and the paddles.

Two positions are recommended for the placement of defibrillation electrodes. The specific placement recommendations will assure that the maximum amount of electricity will flow through the myocardium. These positions include the anterior apex placement (see Fig. 15-3) and the anterior-posterior placement. The anterior apex placement is more commonly used simply because it is the easier of the two, especially during a cardiac arrest event. With the anterior apex placement, the negative electrode is placed to the right of the sternum, just beneath the clavicle, and the positive electrode is placed to the left of the nipple of the left thorax in the midaxillary position. The anterior-posterior placement positions the anterior or negative electrode over the left precordium, with the posterior or positive electrode in the infrascapular space of the left scapula. Both placement positions have proven equally effective in enhancing the amount of energy that reaches the heart muscle.

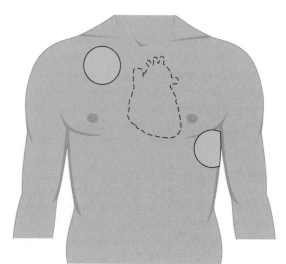

Figure 15-3 Anterior apex placement of defibrillation electrodes.

It is necessary to use some type of commercially available gel pad or electrode gel to eliminate the resistance between the bare chest and the dry metal electrode. Arcing between paddles (caused by contact between the media of each paddle) is a potentially dangerous complication of improperly performed defibrillation. Therefore, only the necessary amount of gel should be used with each paddle.

Another important aspect of successful defibrillation is contact pressure. You should attempt to apply approximately 25 pounds of muscle pressure to ensure good contact of the paddle with the conductive medium against the chest. In addition, this will help to eliminate the chance of arcing of the electrical current. If you are uncertain how much pressure equals 25 pounds, you may press on a standard bathroom scale to achieve 25 pounds on the display. Although this is a rough estimate, it will give you some idea of the amount of pressure needed to equal 25 pounds. Only the muscular strength of your arms should be used.

Table 15-5 depicts the suggested steps that you should follow to correctly perform defibrillation.

If the defibrillation is accomplished in the prehospital field, you should now immediately transfer your patient to the definitive care facility, maintaining constant contact with your Medical Control physician. Be very careful and specific with your documentation of the event.

CARDIOVERSION

Remember that at all times your patient's clinical condition will dictate the care that you render as an emergency health care provider. Keeping that important fact in mind, you should maintain constant vigilance of the patient's appearance, as well as his/her vital signs [level of consciousness

---

TABLE 15-5 PROCEDURE FOR DEFIBRILLATION

Step 1: Be sure to confirm VF or pulseless VT on the cardiac monitor.

Step 2: Assure that the patient is in a safe location (not surrounded by metal or water).

Step 3: Apply electrode gel to paddles or defibrillator pads and to the patient's exposed chest.

Step 4: Turn on and charge the defibrillator to 200 joules for the initial shock.

Step 5: Ensure that the electrodes are in proper position and that proper pressure is applied.

Step 6: Call "Clear." LOOK, SAY, AND SEE CLEAR. Assure that no one is in contact with the patient.

Step 7: Deliver the shock by depressing both red buttons simultaneously (button color and placement may vary depending on manufacturer).

Step 8: Reconfirm the rhythm on the monitor; if VF/VT persists, recharge and repeat steps 5–7 using higher energy levels.

(LOC), pulse rate, respiratory rate, blood pressure]. In the emergent setting, you must determine whether your patient is perfusing, as evidenced by the presence of a pulse. It is also imperative that you diligently monitor the patient's EKG pattern.

Indications for emergency synchronized cardioversion are patient dependent and include perfusing ventricular tachycardia that is unstable or unresponsive to drug therapy, paroxysmal supraventricular tachycardia, and, in some cases, rapid atrial fibrillation. If your patient's condition is hemodynamically unstable, as evidenced by an altered level of consciousness or a decreasing blood pressure, and the cardiac monitor is showing evidence of ventricular tachycardia (with a palpable pulse) or paroxysmal supraventricular tachycardia, then cardioversion should be initiated. Cardioversion should be accomplished following the placement of an IV lifeline and the administration of oxygen. If time allows, and with permission from Medical Control or attending physician, the patient should be sedated.

Emergency synchronized cardioversion is the delivery of an electrical shock to the heart, synchronized so as to coincide with the R wave of the cardiac cycle, thus avoiding the vulnerable relative refractory period. You will recall that, during the relative refractory period, the myocardial muscle cells may be capable of accepting a stimulus, whereas in the absolute refractory period, no stimulus can be accepted. Synchronized cardioversion is designed to deliver the shock approximately 10 milliseconds after the peak of the R wave of the cardiac cycle.

You will recall that with defibrillation, the operator determines when the energy will be delivered. However, with synchronized cardioversion, the exact time of the delivery of electrical current is very specific. The process of synchronization reduces the energy required to terminate dysrhythmias.

Energy requirements for synchronized cardioversion are based on the type of dysrhythmia being treated. Certain dysrhythmias—notably those of atrial origin—can be treated with as little as 10 joules. Most often, if the dysrhythmia is atrial is origin, you should elect to use an initial energy setting of 50 joules. If the dysrhythmia appears to be ventricular in origin, it is recommended that the initial energy setting be 100 joules. You should always follow your local protocol and allow Medical Control to guide your treatment regime.

Procedure for Cardioversion

You will note that, when the defibrillator is placed in the synchronized mode, the EKG displayed on the oscilloscope shows a marker denoting where in the cardiac cycle the energy will be discharged. The marker should appear on the R wave of the QRS complex. If the marker does not appear, you must adjust the EKG size until the marker appears atop the R wave or switch to a different lead that depicts a positively deflected R wave. Table 15-6 illustrates the steps to be followed during synchronized cardioversion.

If the cardioversion was performed in the prehospital field, you should now immediately transfer your patient to the definitive care facility, maintaining constant contact with your Medical Control physician. Again, it is important that you carefully and precisely document the event.

TABLE 15-6 PROCEDURE FOR SYNCHRONIZED CARDIOVERSION

Step 1: Confirm the presence of appropriate rhythm on the cardiac monitor.

Step 2: Assure that the patient is in a safe location (not surrounded by metal or water).

Step 3: Apply electrode gel to paddles or defibrillator pads and to the patient's exposed chest.

Step 4: Turn on the defibrillator, select synchronization mode, and set the proper energy level.

Step 5: Ensure that electrodes are in proper position and that proper pressure is applied.

Step 6: Call "Clear." LOOK, SAY, AND SEE CLEAR. Assure that no one is in contact with the patient.

Step 7: Deliver the shock by depressing both red buttons simultaneously and holding until the unit discharges.

Step 8: Reconfirm the rhythm on the monitor; if the rhythm persists, recharge and repeat steps 5–7 using higher energy levels.

REVIEW QUESTIONS: CHAPTER 15

1. The goal of management of the patient with symptomatic chest pain is to attempt to:
   a. Administer prehospital thrombolytics
   b. Stop the infarction process
   c. Reverse the infarction process
   d. Alleviate the patient's symptoms

2. The maximum benefit of thrombolytic therapy is best achieved when the agent is administered within _____ hours after onset of symptoms.
   a. 2
   b. 10
   c. 6
   d. 1

3. The most commonly utilized tool to indicate the presence of myocardial damage that may lead to infarction is:
   a. ST segment depression
   b. ST segment elevation
   c. Pathologic Q wave
   d. Prolonged PR Interval

4. The major complication of thrombolytic therapy is:

a. Urticaria

b. Thrombosis

c. Dysrhythmia

d. Hemorrhage

5. All of the following clinical presentations may indicate the need for thrombolytic therapy except:

a. Pallor

b. Diaphoresis

c. Ventricular fibrillation

d. Chest pain unrelieved by rest

6. Inclusion criteria for thrombolytic therapy include all of the following except:

a. Age less than 75 years

b. Onset of chest pain occurring within 12 hr

c. Most benefit from thrombolysis if given within 6 hr

d. ST segment elevation $\geq$ 1 mm in 3 or more contiguous limb leads

7. External cardiac pacing (TCP) is sometimes indicated for the treatment of certain reperfusion dysrhythmias, such as:

a. Asymptomatic bradycardia

b. Symptomatic bradycardia

c. Asymptomatic tachycardia

d. Symptomatic tachycardia

8. One of the more common complications of transcutaneous pacing is:

a. Pain

b. Burns

c. Electrocution

d. Muscle damage

9. There are many factors that may determine the amount of transthoracic resistance to current flow. These factors include all of the following except:

a. Room temperature

b. Electrode size

c. Energy level selection

d. Electrode position

10. In the emergent setting, you must determine whether your patient is perfusing, as evidenced by the presence of a:

a. Pulse

b. Heart rhythm

c. Heart rate

d. Blood pressure

11. Synchronized cardioversion is designed to deliver the shock approximately 10 milliseconds after the peak of the _____ wave of the cardiac cycle.

a. Q

b. R

c. S

d. P

12. Energy requirements for synchronized cardioversion are based on the:

a. Number of QRS complexes in a 6-sec strip

b. Type of dysrhythmia being treated

c. Defibrillator capacity

d. Manufacturer's guidelines

16

CARDIOVASCULAR PHARMACOLOGY

Objectives

Upon completion of this chapter, the student will be able to:

1. Explain the drug known as oxygen
2. Describe and list the indications, precautions, side effects, contraindications, and dosages for oxygen
3. Discuss the class of drugs known as sympathomimetics
4. Describe and list the indications, precautions, side effects, contraindications, and dosages for epinephrine, isoproterenol, dopamine, and amrinone
5. Explain the class of drugs known as sympatholytics
6. Describe and list the indications, precautions, side effects, contraindications, and dosages for beta blockers
7. Explain the class of drugs known as antidysrhythmics
8. Describe and list the indications, precautions, side effects, contraindications, and dosages for lidocaine, procainamide, amiodarone, bretylium, atropine sulfate, adenosine, verapamil, and digitalis
9. Discuss the class of drugs known as analgesics
10. Describe and list the indications, precautions, side effects, contraindications, and dosages for morphine sulfate and meperidine
11. Explain the class of drugs known as antianginals
12. Describe and list the indications, precautions, side effects, contraindications, and dosages for nitroglycerin
13. Explain the class of drugs known as alkalinizing agents
14. Describe and list the indications, precautions, side effects, contraindications, and dosages for sodium bicarbonate
15. Explain the class of drugs known as anticoagulants
16. Describe and list the indications, precautions, side effects, contraindications, and dosages for heparin

Pharmacological therapy is an essential component of the overall treatment and care of the patient who may be experiencing an acute myocardial infarction. In addition, the frequency of the occurrence of reperfusion dysrhythmias that are encountered as a result of thrombolytic therapy dictates that the health care provider must be knowledgeable in the area of cardiovascular pharmacology.

Throughout this text, and in the companion book, *Understanding EKGs: A Practical Approach,* we have repeatedly stressed to you the importance of quality patient care. In this chapter, we will discuss the pharmacological components that you will utilize in your care and treatment of patients who are or may be experiencing acute myocardial infarction. Just as observing your patient's clinical condition is a MUST when administering thrombolytic agents, you must also be diligent in your observation of the patient who has received a pharmacological agent. You must question whether the drug administered has had the desired effect, as well as whether your patient's overall condition has improved as a result of the pharmacological agent that was administered.

The following drugs are among the most commonly used cardiovascular pharmacological agents. You should take the time required to study and learn the drugs listed in this chapter. When you, as a health care provider, are in an emergent situation, you will often be a key team member (or perhaps a team leader). In order for you to be comfortable in this role, your knowledge level must continually be heightened and refreshed. We have thus elected to conclude the content of this text with the pharmacological agents that you will most commonly encounter in your management of the patient who is receiving thrombolytic therapy.

We believe that the presentation of this particular subject can initially be a bit overwhelming. Consequently, we have chosen to present the pharmacologic agents in a simple, straightforward, and specific format. Each agent is discussed within its specific classification. We will then briefly discuss the most important aspects of each agent, namely, the mechanisms of action, indications, precautions, side effects, contraindications, and dosages.

OXYGEN

The "drug" that is most often used and whose importance **cannot** be overemphasized is oxygen. We are well aware that you have read and heard that statement numerous times; however, it is a vital component of emergency cardiac care that must never be forgotten or overlooked. Oxygen is a colorless, odorless, tasteless gas that is absolutely necessary to sustain life.

Mechanism of Action
Oxygen rapidly circulates across the alveolar walls and attaches to hemoglobin molecules in the red blood cells. During the process of systemic circulation, oxygen is distributed throughout the body to achieve adequate tissue perfusion. Oxygen is essential for the body to maintain its normal metabolic activities. Metabolism that occurs in the absence of oxygen is

termed **anaerobic** metabolism. The end product of anaerobic metabolism is lactic acid, which, in combination with increased carbon dioxide levels, will lead to respiratory and metabolic acidoses. It is for this reason that proper oxygenation of body cells is so critical.

Indications

- Hypoxia, secondary to trauma or illness

Precautions

- Chronic obstructive pulmonary disease (COPD)

Side Effects

- Oxygen toxicity
- Epistaxis, in prolonged administration of nonhumidified oxygen

Contraindications

- None, in the emergent situation

Dosage

- Based on the patient's clinical condition
- In the emergent situation, 100% oxygen is usually administered

SYMPATHOMIMETICS

Sympathomimetics are agents that mimic the actions of the sympathetic nervous system (see Fig. 16-1). These agents either directly or indirectly stimulate the sympathetic nervous system. As a result, hormones called catecholamines are released within the body. The subsequent result is an increase in sympathetic tone that ultimately leads to an increase in heart rate and myocardial contractility.

For the purposes of this chapter, we will primarily discuss information that relates to the effects of cardiovascular pharmacological agents as well as to the patients who are treated as a result of cardiac disorders.

Epinephrine

Mechanism of Action

Epinephrine is a naturally occurring catecholamine that acts to stimulate both the alpha- and beta-adrenergic receptor sites. At this point, you may wish to refer to page 13 in the companion book to refresh your knowledge of the autonomic nervous system. The stimulation of these receptor sites increases the activity of the heart and dilates the bronchioles.

Cardiac Effects Include

- Increased heart rate
- Increased contractility

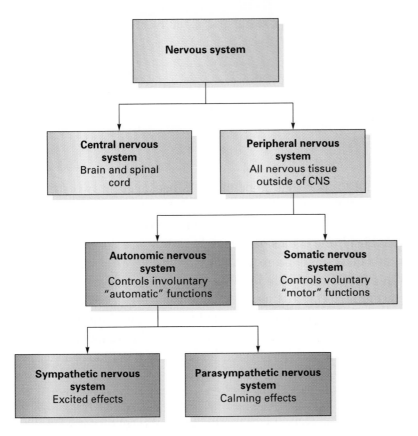

Figure 16-1 Nervous system components.

- Increased activity of the electrical conduction system
- Increased systemic vascular resistance

Indications
- Management of cardiac arrest
- Severe anaphylaxis

In the emergent setting, the administration of epinephrine can convert asystole to fine ventricular fibrillation (V-fib) and can convert fine V-fib to coarse V-fib. As we discussed earlier in this chapter, the chance of successful defibrillation is enhanced by administration of epinephrine and proper oxygenation.

Precautions
- Can be deactivated if mixed with alkaline agents; the intravenous (IV) line should be flushed prior to and following the administration of sodium bicarbonate
- Should be protected from light

Side Effects
- May create dysrhythmias secondary to increased workload of the heart
- Increased myocardial oxygen demand

- Anxiety, nervousness, restlessness, tachycardia, headache
- Hypertension

Contraindications

- In the face of severe cardiovascular compromise, there are no absolute contraindications

Dosage

It is important to note that epinephrine is packaged in two strengths. The common packaging for intravenous administration yields 1 milligram of epinephrine in 10 milliliters of solution (1:10,000) in a prefilled syringe. In addition, epinephrine comes packaged for intramuscular (IM), endotracheal (ET), or subcutaneous administration in a solution of 1:1,000 or 1 milligram of drug in 1 milliliter of solution. The latter of these two solutions is much more concentrated (more drug, less solution). Certain enzymes in the body constantly degrade epinephrine, consequently decreasing the effects of the drug. For this reason, it is necessary to administer frequent doses. Current research indicates that high-dose epinephrine (HDE) may have beneficial effects in the cardiac arrest state.

- Cardiac arrest
  —1 milligram every 3 to 5 minutes via IV push or via ET tube; utilize 1:10,000 solution
  —Consider high-dose epinephrine if the traditional doses have proved ineffective following numerous attempts. Escalating-dose epinephrine administration is typically initiated at a dosage of 1, 3, or 5 milligrams 3 to 5 minutes apart. However, you should always follow local protocol, as well as Medical Direction.
- Anaphylaxis
  —0.3 to 0.5 milligrams of a 1:1,000 solution, administered subcutaneously
  —Repeat same dose every 5 to 15 minutes

Isoproterenol (Isuprel)

Mechanism of Action

Isoproterenol primarily acts on beta-adrenergic receptors. This drug is a synthetic catecholamine. Isuprel produces an overall increase in heart rate and myocardial contractility. It promotes vasodilation and relaxation of the pulmonary bronchioles. This drug is used in cardiac emergency situations to increase heart rate in bradycardias that are refractory to atropine. The existence of transcutaneous cardiac pacing (TCP) and of other drugs that have fewer side effects has rendered Isuprel less popular than was once the case.

Indications

- Bradycardias resulting from high-degree heart blocks (second-degree Mobitz Type II and third-degree blocks), especially when TCP is unavailable

- Bradycardias refractory to atropine, when TCP is not available

Precautions
- Increased myocardial oxygen demands
- Patient should be continually monitored for signs of ventricular irritability, such as premature ventricular contractions (PVCs), ventricular tachycardia (V-tach), or even V-fib
- Can be deactivated by alkaline solutions (sodium bicarbonate)
- Should be used cautiously in patients with digitalis toxicity as it may exacerbate tachydysrhythmias

Side Effects
- Myocardial ischemia
- Hypokalemia (decreased potassium level)
- Hypertension
- Tremor, tachycardia, restlessness, nervousness

Contraindications
- Cardiogenic shock
- Not recommended for use as a first-line drug for the treatment of brady-dysrhythmias in the hemodynamically unstable patient

Dosage
- Administered via IV infusion (utilize mini-drip set) by mixing 1 milligram of Isuprel in 250 cubic centimeters of D5W; mixture yields 4 micrograms per cubic centimeter; administer 2 to 10 micrograms per minute, titrated to desired hemodynamic effect [heart rate (HR) 60 beats per minute (BPM) or systolic blood pressure (BP) 90 or above]

Dopamine (Intropin)

Mechanism of Action
Dopamine is a naturally occurring catecholamine that is a chemical precursor of norepinephrine. Dopamine acts on alpha-, beta-, and dopaminergic adrenergic receptors. This drug promotes vasoconstriction and increases myocardial contractility. The effect of this drug depends directly upon the amount administered.

Indications
- Nonhypovolemic hypotension
- Cardiogenic shock

Precautions
- Increases heart rate
- Can worsen supraventricular and ventricular dysrhythmias

- Must be discontinued if tachydysrhythmias or ventricular fibrillation develop

Side Effects

- Hypokalemia
- Development of dysrhythmias
- Nausea, vomiting, tachycardia, restlessness, nervousness

Contraindications

- Never used as a first-line or single agent in the management of hypovolemic shock unless fluid resuscitation is well under way
- Should not be used in patients with known pheochromocytoma (tumor of the adrenal glands)

Dosage

- Mix 800 milligrams of dopamine in 500 cubic centimeters D5W; mixture yields 1,600 micrograms per cubic centimeter
- Renal dose: 2–5 micrograms per kilogram per minute; renal output greatly increased
- Cardiac dose: 5–10 micrograms per kilogram per minute; increase in cardiac output and BP
- Vasopressor dose: 10–20 micrograms per kilogram per minute; increase in blood pressure

Amrinone (Inocor)

Mechanism of Action

Inocor is a rapidly acting positive inotropic agent. An inotropic agent is an agent that affects contractility or force. A positive inotropic agent increases contractility, whereas a negative inotropic agent decreases contractility. This drug increases vasodilation and consequently decreases the workload of the heart. Inocor is helpful when there is fluid in the pulmonary vessels and lung fields because it improves myocardial output.

Indications

- Congestive heart failure refractory to diuretics and vasodilators or severe left ventricular dysfunction

Precautions

- Increased myocardial ischemia
- Due to chemical incompatibility, Inocor should not be diluted in solutions containing dextrose
- Lasix should not be administered in an IV line delivering Inocor, as precipitates will form due to chemical incompatibilities

Side Effects

- May cause dysrhythmias, hypotension, nausea, vomiting
- May cause thrombocytopenia (decreased platelets)

Contraindications

- Sensitivity to sulfur compounds
- Should not be used as a first-line agent in congestive heart failure (CHF) or left ventricular failure (LVF)

Dosage

- Therapy should be initiated with an IV bolus (loading dose) of 0.75 milligrams per kilogram over a period of 2 to 5 minutes
- Follow with an infusion prepared with 100 milligrams mixed into 500 cubic centimeters of normal saline; mixture yields 0.2 milligrams per cubic centimeter
- Maintenance infusion of 2 to 5 micrograms per kilogram per minute

SYMPATHOLYTICS

Beta Blockers

Mechanism of Action

Beta blockers antagonize (oppose) adrenergic receptor sites. In simpler terms, beta blockers obstruct the receptor site and serve to prevent or inhibit stimulation; this action produces effects such as slowed conduction impulses and decreased heart rate and contractility.

Indications

- Used to control recurrent ventricular fibrillation, ventricular tachycardia, or paroxysmal supraventricular tachycardia (PSVT)
- Long-term treatment of myocardial infarction by decreasing the overall workload of the heart and myocardial oxygen consumption

Precautions

- Can precipitate serious bronchospasm; should be used with caution in patients with history of COPD, asthma, or CHF
- May decrease heart rate to unacceptable levels

Side Effects

- Hypotension secondary to decreased heart rate and contractility
- Pulmonary congestion secondary to bronchodilation

Contraindications

- Preexisting bradycardia
- COPD, asthma
- CHF

Dosages

- Atenolol (Tenormin)
  —IV administration: 5-milligram IV push over 5 minutes
  —Same dosage repeated 10 minutes later if needed
  —Oral dosing should begin 10 minutes after second IV dose (50 milligrams)
- Metoprolol (Lopressor)
  —5-milligram IV push over 2 to 5 minutes
  —Readminister two times at 5-minute intervals, not to exceed 15 milligrams total
  —Oral administration following IV dosing should range between 180 and 300 milligrams daily
- Propranolol (Inderal)
  —For IV administration, 1- to 3-milligram IV push over 2 to 5 minutes
  —Can be repeated after 2 minutes, to a total dose of 0.1 milligram per kilogram

ANTIDYSRHYTHMICS

The general classification of drugs that serve to remedy disturbances in the heart's electrical activity are known as **antidysrhythmics.** If, for example, a patient's heart rate becomes too fast or too slow, the physician may choose to prescribe an antidysrhythmic. In addition, antidysrhythmics may be used to correct disruptions in cardiac conduction.

Lidocaine

Mechanism of Action
The mechanisms of action of lidocaine are numerous. The more commonly recognized mechanisms of action of this agent include:

- Depresses depolarization and automaticity in the ventricles
- Suppresses ventricular ectopy (out-of-place) rhythm in the setting of myocardial infarction
- Increases ventricular fibrillation threshold (*threshold* refers to a point at which a stimulus will produce a cell response)
- Does not affect myocardial contractility or conduction of the sino-atrial (SA) or atrioventricular (AV) nodes

Indications
- Lidocaine is the drug of choice in the treatment of dysrhythmias that are a result of ventricular irritability, specifically:
  —Ventricular tachycardia
  —Ventricular fibrillation
- Suppression of malignant premature ventricular contractions (PVCs), that is:
  —More than six PVCs per minute

—Multifocal PVCs
—Couplet PVCs
—R-on-T phenomenon

Precautions

- Depressed liver function (delay in removing lidocaine from the body)
- Central nervous system depression (decreased level of consciousness, irritability, confusion, eventual seizures)

Side Effects

- Drowsiness
- Bradycardia, heart block, cardiac arrest
- Respiratory arrest
- Hypoxia
- Nausea and vomiting

Contraindications

- Second-degree, Type II, and infranodal heart blocks
- Bradycardia with PVCs (PVCs may be the body's attempt to maintain cardiac perfusion; abolishing these PVCs with lidocaine can lead to cardiac arrest)
- Lidocaine sensitivity

Dosage

- Administer 1 to 1.5 milligrams per kilogram via IV bolus (in ET administration, give 2 to 2.5 mg/kg)
- Place 2 grams in 500 cubic centimeters D5W or normal saline; infuse at a rate of 30 gtt per minute using a minidrip set (60-microgtt set), which will yield 2 milligrams per minute, and titrate (slowly change rate of administration) to desired effect (until PVCs are suppressed). If using an IV pump with a standard set, you should reference the specific pump recommendations.
- Second dose should be decreased by 50% with geriatric patients

Procainamide

Mechanism of Action

In cases where lidocaine has not proven effective or in cases of lidocaine sensitivity, procainamide may prove effective in the suppression of ventricular ectopies. In addition, it is important to understand that procainamide reduces the automaticity of the various pacemaker sites in the heart, as well as slowing intraventricular conduction to a much greater degree than does lidocaine.

Indications

- Ventricular dysrhythmias refractory to lidocaine; that is, persistent malignant PVCs, persistent ventricular tachycardia with a pulse, persistent ventricular fibrillation/pulseless ventricular tachycardia

Precautions

- Bradycardia with PVCs
- Should be used with caution in the hypotensive patient
- Should be discontinued if QRS complex widens by more than 50% from pretreatment width
- Should not exceed maximum dose of 17 milligrams per kilogram

Side Effects

- Drowsiness, confusion
- Hypersensitivity
- Seizures
- Hypotension, bradycardia, heart blocks
- Nausea and vomiting

Contraindications

- Should not be administered to patients with severe conduction system disturbances, especially second- and third-degree heart blocks
- Profound hypotension (<80 mmHg systolic)

Dosage

- Administer 1 gram in 50 milliliters of D5W (20 mg/ml) at a rate of 20 to 30 milligrams per minute, until maximum dose of 17 milligrams per kilogram, followed by:
- Maintenance infusion of 1 gram in 500 milliliters D5W, which equals a 2:1 ratio; begin by administering 15 gtt per minute and titrate to effect

Amiodarone (Cordarone)

Mechanism of Action

Amiodarone prolongs the refractory period of the myocardial cells. In addition, this agent causes systemic vasodilation. The primary therapeutic effect of amiodarone is the suppression of dysrhythmias.

Indications

- Management of life-threatening ventricular dysrhythmias unresponsive to primary antidysrhythmic agents
- Recurring ventricular fibrillation
- Hemodynamically stable or unstable ventricular tachycardia

Precautions

- History of congestive heart failure
- Severe pulmonary or liver disease

Side Effects

- Headache

- Bradycardia
- Hypotension

Contraindications

- Known hypersensitivity
- Should not be administered to patients with severe conduction system disturbances, especially second- and third-degree heart blocks
- Profound hypotension (<80 mmHg systolic)

Dosage

- Administer 150 milligrams (3 ml) IV over a 10-minute period; add 150 milligrams to 100 cubic centimeters D5W to equal 1.5 milligrams per milliliter
- Infusion: add 900 milligrams to 500 milliliters D5W (concentration of 1.8 mg/ml): slowly administer 360 milligrams over the next 6 hours at 1 milligram per minute
- Dosage for V-fib/pulseless VT is 150 milligrams in 50 cubic centimeters D5W over 15 to 30 seconds

Bretylium Tosylate

Mechanism of Action

Bretylium is generally not considered a first-line agent in the treatment of dysrhythmias.

Bretylium causes two effects on adrenergic nerve endings. Initially, this agent causes release of norepinephrine, resulting in a slight increase in heart rate, blood pressure, and cardiac output. These initial effects last approximately 20 minutes. Then norepinephrine release is inhibited, resulting in hypotension. The exact effect of bretylium is poorly understood, but it appears that the agent elevates the ventricular fibrillation threshold in much the same way as lidocaine.

Indications

- Persistent malignant PVCs
- Ventricular fibrillation refractory to lidocaine
- Ventricular tachycardia refractory to lidocaine

Precautions

- Since postural hypotension occurs in approximately 50% of patients who receive bretylium, this side effect should be anticipated; therefore, keep patient supine

Side Effects

- Dizziness, syncope, seizures
- Hypotension

- Hypertension
- Angina
- Nausea and vomiting

Contraindications
- None, when used in the treatment of life-threatening ventricular dysrhythmias

Dosage
- Administer 5-milligram per kilogram IV push over 8 to 10 minutes
- Second dose 10-milligram per kilogram IV push
- Subsequent doses may be administered every 10 minutes, not to exceed 30 milligrams per kilogram
- Infusion: 1 gram in 500 cubic centimeters D5W or normal saline; yields 2-milligram per milliliter concentration; initiate infusion of 1 milligram per minute utilizing microdrip set; infuse at 30 microgtt per minute

Atropine Sulfate

Mechanism of Action

Atropine is classified further as a rate-control antidysrhythmic, as well as a parasympatholytic (an agent that blocks the effects of the parasympathetic nervous system). Atropine increases the heart rate by blocking vagal tone (parasympathetic reduction in heart rate).

Indications
- Hemodynamically unstable (symptomatic) bradycardia
- Asystole

Precautions
- Maximum dose should not exceed 0.04 milligrams per kilogram
- Use with caution in patients who present with third-degree block
- Be prepared to artificially pace the patient

Side Effects
- Blurred vision
- Dry mouth
- Dilation of the pupils
- Tachycardia
- Drowsiness and confusion

Contraindications
- Hypersensitivity
- Tachycardia

Dosage

- 0.5- to 1-milligram IV push (if administered via ET tube, 1 to 2 mg)
- Repeat dose every 3 to 5 minutes, to a maximum dose of 0.04 milligrams per kilogram

Adenosine

Mechanism of Action

Adenosine works to interrupt reentry pathways in the AV node and slows conduction time through the AV node. This agent also produces coronary artery vasodilation and thus enhances myocardial perfusion.

Indications

- Symptomatic PSVT
- Wide complex tachycardia of unknown etiology

Precautions

- Hypersensitivity
- Use cautiously in patients with histories of unstable angina or asthma
- Effects may be decreased by theophylline or caffeine

Side Effects

- Transient dysrhythmias
- Facial flushing
- Nausea, dyspnea
- Headache
- Chest pain, palpitations, and hypotension

Contraindications

- Hypersensitivity
- Second- or third-degree heart block

Dosage

- 6-milligram rapid IV bolus over 1 to 2 seconds; wait 1 to 2 minutes, then give 12-milligram rapid IV bolus over 1 to 2 seconds; may consider third dose
- Total dose not to exceed 30 milligrams

Verapamil (Isoptin, Calan)

Mechanism of Action

Verapamil is a calcium channel blocker. Calcium channel blockers relax vascular smooth muscle, cause vascular dilation, and consequently act to slow conduction through the AV node. Verapamil also serves to reduce myocardial oxygen demand, while at the same time inhibiting dysrhythmias that are secondary to reentry, such as PSVT.

Indications

- PSVT refractory to adenosine

Precautions

- May cause systemic hypotension; BP must be monitored vigilantly

Side Effects

- Nausea and vomiting
- Dizziness
- Headache
- Tachycardia
- Hypotension
- Heart block and asystole

Contraindications

- Should not be administered to patients with severe hypotension
- Cardiogenic shock
- Should not be administered in the prehospital arena to patients with ventricular tachycardia
- Wolff-Parkinson-White syndrome

Dosage

- In PSVT, initial dosage is 2.5- to 5-milligram IV push over a 2- to 3-minute interval
- Repeat dosage of 5 to 10 milligrams can be given over a 15- to 30-minute period if PSVT persists and the patient has demonstrated no adverse effects
- Total dose should not exceed 30 milligrams in 30 minutes

Digitalis (Digoxin, Lanoxin)

Mechanism of Action

Digitalis is a cardiac glycoside that increases the force of cardiac contraction, as well as cardiac output. This agent slows impulse conduction through the AV node. The administration of digitalis serves to decrease the ventricular response to certain supraventricular dysrhythmias such as paroxysmal supraventricular tachycardia, atrial flutter, and atrial fibrillation.

Indications

- Congestive heart failure
- PSVT
- Atrial fibrillation
- Atrial flutter

Precautions

- Patients require constant monitoring for signs and symptoms of digitalis toxicity
- Should not be given to a patient with a heart rate of less than 60 BPM
- Use cautiously in patients with documented electrolyte imbalances

Side Effects

- Digitalis toxicity (yellow vision, nausea, vomiting, drowsiness, new-onset heart blocks)
- Dysrhythmias

Contraindications

Lanoxin should not be administered to patients who:

- Are in ventricular fibrillation
- Show any of the signs or symptoms of digitalis toxicity
- Show evidence of heart blocks

Dosage

- Initial IV dose: 0.6 to 1 milligram at 4- to 8-hour intervals
- Initial oral dose: 0.75 to 1.25 milligrams

ANALGESICS

Morphine Sulfate (Morphine, MS)

Mechanism of Action

Morphine sulfate is classified as a narcotic analgesic. In fact, this agent is one of the most potent analgesics on the market. MS is a central nervous system depressant that has hemodynamic properties that make it quite useful in the field of emergency medicine.

Indications

- Pulmonary edema (with or without associated pain)
- Severe chest pain associated with myocardial infarction
- Severe pain associated with kidney stones

Precautions

- Tendency for abuse and addiction
- In high doses, may cause severe respiratory depression
- Narcotic antagonists (such as Narcan) should be immediately available when this agent is administered
- This agent is a controlled substance and must be kept in a locked cabinet or drug bag

Side Effects

- Nausea and vomiting
- Blurred vision
- Pupillary constriction
- Altered mental status
- Headache
- Respiratory depression

Contraindications

- Hypersensitivity
- Should not be administered to volume-depleted patients
- Should not be administered to severely hypotensive patients

Dosage

- Initial dose of 2- to 10-milligram slow IV push, titrated to effect
- Additional doses of 2 milligrams IV may be administered every few minutes until pain is relieved

Meperidine (Demerol)

Mechanism of Action

Meperidine is classified as a narcotic analgesic. This agent is a central nervous system depressant that is widely used in medicine in the treatment of moderate to severe pain. Although meperidine is a potent analgesic, it is not as potent as morphine sulfate. Also, the rate of onset of this agent is slightly faster than that of morphine, yet its effects are much shorter in duration.

Indications

- Moderate to severe pain

Precautions

- May cause respiratory distress
- Narcan should always be available to reverse the effects of the drug if respiratory depression ensues
- This agent is a controlled substance and must be kept in a locked cabinet or drug bag

Side Effects

- Nausea and vomiting
- Abdominal cramps
- Blurred vision
- Constricted pupils
- Altered mental status, headache, hallucinations
- Respiratory depression

Contraindications

- Hypersensitivity
- Should not be administered to patients with undiagnosed abdominal pain or head injury

Dosage

- Initial dose for treatment of severe pain is 25 to 50 milligrams IV
- Standard dose is 50 to 100 milligrams IM; however, when dealing with cardiac patients, IM injections should be avoided due to the effects on cardiac enzyme levels
- Often administered with an antiemetic agent due to its tendency to cause nausea/vomiting

ANTIANGINALS

Nitroglycerin (Nitrostat)

Mechanism of Action

Nitroglycerin is a powerful smooth muscle relaxant and is often used in the treatment of angina pectoris. Because of the relaxant properties of this agent, it can drastically reduce preload and cardiac workload. This agent also dilates coronary arteries, resulting in an increase in coronary blood flow. Consequently, the perfusion of the compromised myocardial muscle is increased. As the ischemia of the myocardial cells is alleviated, the patient will report a decrease in the intensity of his/her chest pain. If indeed the patient's chest pain was caused by myocardial ischemia, the administration of nitroglycerin will generally minimize the pain within 1 to 3 minutes following the dosage.

Indications

- Chest pain associated with angina pectoris
- Chest pain associated with acute myocardial infarction
- Acute pulmonary edema (unless accompanied by hypotension)

Precautions

- Development of tolerance to the drug may necessitate increased dosages
- Drug rapidly deteriorates after the bottle is opened
- Must be protected from light
- Blood pressure and all vital signs should be closely monitored

Side Effects

- Headaches are common following the administration of this agent, as a result of cerebral vasodilation
- Dizziness, weakness
- Tachycardia and hypotension

- Dry mouth
- Nausea and vomiting

Contraindications
- Hypotension
- Increased intracranial pressure
- Shock

Dosage
- For angina pectoris, initial dose is 1 tablet (0.4 mg) sublingually
- Dose may be repeated in 3 to 5 minutes as required
- In the prehospital setting, no more than three tablets should be administered
- Agent is also available in spray, ointment, and patch forms
- May be administered IV in the emergency department or intensive care unit setting or during intrafacility transfers

ALKALINIZING AGENTS

Sodium Bicarbonate

Mechanism of Action
Sodium bicarbonate is an alkalinizing agent that is sometimes utilized in the treatment of metabolic acidosis. This drug is a salt that provides bicarbonate to serve as a buffer in the management of metabolic acidosis. It is also used in the treatment of tricyclic antidepressant overdose to cause urine to be more alkaline by raising the pH and consequently to speed the excretion of urine.

Indications
- May be used in the treatment of cardiac arrest in documented cases of metabolic acidosis
- Tricyclic antidepressant overdose
- Severe acidosis refractory to hyperventilation
- Phenobarbital overdose

Precautions
- When administered in large doses, may produce metabolic alkalosis
- Should not be administered in conjunction with calcium chloride, as a precipitate can form and lead to clogging of the IV line

Side Effects
- Metabolic alkalosis
- Few when administered in the emergent setting

Contraindications

- No absolute contraindication

Dosage

- Should be administered only by IV bolus
- Initial dose: 1 milliequivalent per kilogram of body weight, followed by 0.5 milliequivalent per kilogram every 10 minutes
- Whenever possible, dosage should be guided by arterial blood gas studies

ANTICOAGULANTS

Heparin

Mechanism of Action

Heparin is classified as an anticoagulant and is often used in conjunction with certain thrombolytic agents. It may also be used after thrombolysis (*thrombo* = clot, *lysis* = dissolve) has occurred. In simpler terms, heparin increases the length of time required for clots to reform.

Indications

- Given in conjunction with thrombolytic surgery
- Pulmonary embolus

Precautions

- Severe liver disease
- Severe kidney disease
- Risk of bleeding increased when administered in conjunction with aspirin or nonsteroidal anti-inflammatory drugs

Side Effects

- Allergic reactions
- Bruising
- Epistaxis
- Hematuria

Contraindications

- Presence of active bleeding
- Severe hypotension
- Recent intracranial surgery
- Hypersensitivity

Dosage

- 5,000 to 10,000 units IV push

- Followed by infusion of 1,000 units per hour for 24 to 48 hours (25,000 U in 500 cc D5W at a rate of 10 cc/hr)

REVIEW QUESTIONS: CHAPTER 16

1. Atropine 1.0 milligrams may:
   1. Be given via ET tube
   2. Be useful in third-degree AV block
   3. Result in undesirable heart block
   4. Increase the rate of a sinus bradycardia

   a. 1, 2, 3
   b. 1, 2, 4
   c. 2, 3, 4
   d. 1, 3

2. External pacing may be indicated for the following rhythms when the rhythms are refractory to atropine:
   a. Pulseless electrical activity
   b. First-degree atrioventricular block
   c. Symptomatic bradycardia
   d. Symptomatic ventricular tachycardia

3. An adult weighing 72 kilograms presents with ventricular tachycardia and a palpable pulse. Which of the following schedules of lidocaine is preferred?
   a. IV bolus of 75 mg, followed by infusion at 2–4 mg/min
   b. IV bolus of 150 mg every 5 min to a total of 300 mg
   c. 150-mg IV bolus followed by infusion of 4–6 mg/min
   d. 200-mg IV bolus followed by infusion of 1–2 mg/min

4. Lidocaine may be administered by the following routes:
   a. IV only
   b. ET only
   c. IV or IM
   d. IV, ET, intraosseous

5. Which of the following statements regarding procainamide administration is false?
   a. Administration of this agent should be discontinued if the patient becomes hypotensive
   b. Administration of this agent should be discontinued when 2 g have been delivered
   c. Procainamide is never administered via the ET tube route

    d. Discontinue administration of this agent if the original QRS width has widened by 50% or more

6. Verapamil is an:

    a. Analgesic

    b. Alkalinizer

    c. Antidysrhythmic

    d. Antihypertensive

7. Epinephrine may be administered:

    a. To relieve the pain of angina pectoris

    b. Via direct epicardial injection

    c. By intraosseous injection

    d. Only via the intravenous route

8. Which of the following drugs increases heart rate?

    a. Atropine

    b. Adenosine

    c. Verapamil

    d. Sodium bicarbonate

9. The trade name for dopamine hydrochloride is:

    a. Amiorone

    b. Intropin

    c. Dobutamine

    d. Diazepam

10. The administration of an IV solution by regulating its flow rate based upon observation or desired or undesired effects is called:

    a. Estimation

    b. Titration

    c. Approximation

    d. Calculation

11. The mechanisms of action of Isuprel include:

    1. Increased heart rate

    2. Increased cardiac output

    3. Increased myocardial oxygen consumption

    4. Production of secondary bronchodilation

    a. 1, 2

    b. 3, 4

    c. 2, 3, 4

    d. 1, 2, 3, 4

12. A 66-year-old female weighing 132 pounds requires a bolus of sodium bicarbonate. The bicarbonate should be administered in a 1-milliequivalent per kilogram bolus. How many milliequivalents per kilogram should be administered to this patient?

a. 20

b. 40

c. 60

d. 80

17

MORE REVIEW QUESTIONS

1. Most cardiac dysrhythmias are caused by ischemia secondary to hypoxia; therefore the most appropriate drug to give a patient with any dysrhythmia is:

    a. Oxygen

    b. D5W

    c. Lidocaine

    d. Morphine

2. The fibrous sac covering of the heart, which is in contact with the pleura, is the:

    a. Epicardium

    b. Myocardium

c. Pericardium

d. Endocardium

3. Mr. Young is a 56-year-old male patient who is experiencing crushing chest pain. Immediately after an intravenous (IV) line has been established, Mr. Young becomes apneic and pulseless. During resuscitation, the physician orders sodium bicarbonate and calcium chloride to be administered. After the administration of the sodium bicarbonate, you then realize that you must:

   a. Immediately proceed to administer the calcium chloride

   b. Flush the IV line before administering the calcium chloride

   c. Wait 15 minutes before administering the calcium chloride

   d. Administer magnesium sulfate prior to the calcium chloride bolus

4. The heart ventricle with the thickest myocardium is the:

   a. Right

   b. Left

5. The pulmonic and aortic valves are open during:

   a. Systole

   b. Diastole

6. The large blood vessel that returns deoxygenated blood from the head and neck to the right atrium is called the:

   a. Jugular vein

   b. Carotid artery

   c. Superior vena cava

   d. Inferior vena cava

7. Accepted uses of sodium bicarbonate include:

   a. Severe acidosis

   b. Complete heart block

   c. Multifocal premature ventricular contractions (PVCs)

   d. Atrial flutter

8. The coronary sinus, which opens into the right atrium, allows venous return from the:

   a. Azygos

   b. Pleura

   c. Myocardium

   d. Endocardium

9. The sawtooth pattern is indicative of which of the following rhythms?

   a. Atrial fibrillation

   b. Atrial asystole

   c. Ventricular flutter

   d. Atrial flutter

10. The mitral valve is located between the:

    a. Right and left atrium

    b. Right and left ventricle

    c. Left atrium and left ventricle

    d. Right atrium and right ventricle

11. When dealing with inferior and inferoposterior myocardial infarctions (MIs), the appearance of high-degree atrioventricular (AV) blocks may be present upon admission to the hospital. Examples of high-degree blocks include:

    a. First-degree block

    b. Second-degree Type I block

    c. Third degree block

    d. Wenckebach/Mobitz Type I block

12. Sodium bicarbonate should be administered:

    a. Intravenously

    b. Intraosseously

    c. Intradermally

    d. Endotracheally

13. The QRS waves of all premature complexes are usually 0.10 second or less in duration.

    a. False

    b. True

14. Which of the following is the most appropriate initial setting for defibrillating ventricular fibrillation in an adult?

    a. 400 joules

    b. 200 joules

    c. 1 joule/kg

    d. 20–25 joules/kg

15. A common cardiac drug encountered frequently in patients' homes as an oral medication is:

    a. Bretylium

    b. Prednisone

    c. Penicillin

    d. Digitalis

16. When preparing to defibrillate a patient who presents with ventricular fibrillation, the health care provider should do all the following except:

    a. Check pulses and lead wires

    b. Order all personnel to stand clear

c. Perform cardiopulmonary resuscitation

d. Ensure that the synchronization button is on

17. The most appropriate treatment for uncomplicated acute myocardial infarction is:

a. IV D5W only

b. Oxygen by mask, IV lactated Ringer solution

c. IV D50W, monitor, oxygen

d. IV normal saline, cardiac monitor, oxygen

18. The coronary arteries receive oxygenated blood from the:

a. Aorta

b. Coronary sinus

c. Pulmonary veins

d. Pulmonary arteries

19. IV fluids are administered to cardiac patients primarily in order to:

a. Provide a lifeline

b. Allow oxygen to the brain

c. Keep the patient well hydrated

d. Prevent incipient pump failure

20. EKG leads that record the electrical impulse formation in uninvolved myocardium directly opposite the involved myocardium are termed:

a. Facing leads

b. Viewing leads

c. Reciprocal leads

d. Endocardial leads

21. The chambers of the heart that are thin-walled and pump against low pressure are the:

a. Apex

b. Aorta

c. Atria

d. Ventricles

22. Blood pressure is maintained by cardiac output and:

a. Alveoli

b. Stroke volume

c. Coronary arteries

d. Peripheral resistance

23. The sinoatrial (SA) node is located in the:

a. Right atrium

b. Right ventricle

    c. Purkinje fiber tract

    d. Atrioventricular septum

24. The AV node is located in the:

    a. Right ventricle

    b. Left ventricle

    c. Purkinje fiber tract

    d. Atrioventricular septum

25. The intrinsic firing rate of the AV node is:

    a. 60–100 BPM

    b. 25–35 BPM

    c. 35–45 BPM

    d. 40–60 BPM

26. EKG findings of infarction may occur in a single lead or in a combination of leads.

    a. True

    b. False

27. A sudden (paroxysmal) onset of tachycardia with a stimulus that arises above the AV node refers to:

    a. Sinus arrest

    b. Sinus tachycardia

    c. Sinus dysrhythmia

    d. Supraventricular dysrhythmia

28. Oscilloscopic evidence of ventricular fibrillation can be mimicked by artifact.

    a. True

    b. False

29. Adenosine is a naturally occurring substance present in all body cells. The mechanism of action of adenosine can be described as:

    a. Increasing conduction of the electrical impulse through the AV node

    b. Decreasing conduction of the electrical impulse through the AV node

    c. Increasing conduction of the electrical impulse through the Purkinje network

    d. Increasing conduction of the electrical impulse through the SA node

30. Administration routes for atropine include:

    a. IV only

    b. Endotracheal (ET) only

c. IV, ET, or intraosseous (IO)

d. IV or ET

31. The intrinsic rate of the SA node in the adult is:

   a. 20–60 BPM

   b. 40–80 BPM

   c. 60–100 BPM

   d. 80–100 BPM

32. The electrocardiogram is used to:

   a. Determine cardiac output

   b. Detect valvular dysfunction

   c. Evaluate electrical activity in the heart

   d. Determine whether the heart muscle is contracting

33. The PR Interval should normally be _____ or smaller.

   a. 0.10 sec

   b. 0.12 sec

   c. 0.08 sec

   d. 0.20 sec

34. Defined as "death of the myocardial tissue," a myocardial infarction commonly results from:

   a. Myocardial necrosis

   b. Myocardial injury

   c. Myocardial ischemia

   d. Muscle oxygenation

35. EKG changes that may be anticipated as a result of myocardial ischemia, injury, and/or necrosis of the myocardial tissues include all of the following except:

   a. PR Interval prolongation

   b. ST segment elevation

   c. ST segment depression

   d. Pathologic Q wave

36. The development of the pathologic Q waves often begins within the first 2 hours after the MI and, in most cases, is complete within:

   a. 60 min

   b. 30 min

   c. 24 hr

   d. 48 hr

37. The QRS interval should normally be _____ or smaller.

a. 0.20 sec

b. 0.12 sec

c. 0.18 sec

d. 0.36 sec

38. The upper chambers of the heart are called:

a. Atria

b. Ventricles

c. Septa

d. Branches

39. A sinus rhythm with cyclic variation caused by alterations in the respiratory pattern is:

a. Sinus arrest

b. Sinus tachycardia

c. Sinus dysrhythmia

d. Supraventricular dysrhythmia

40. In the presence of ventricular fibrillation, ineffective countershock attempts might be caused by:

a. The presence of metabolic acidosis

b. Ventricular irritability

c. Inadequate oxygenation

d. All of the above

41. Prior to performing carotid sinus massage, you should do all the following except:

a. Monitor the EKG

b. Ensure that carotid pulses are present

c. Have the patient perform Valsalva maneuver

d. Establish a secure airway by intubating the trachea

42. The QRS complex is produced when the:

a. Ventricles repolarize

b. Ventricles depolarize

c. Ventricles contract

d. Both b and c

43. Most atrial fibrillation waves are not followed by a QRS complex because:

a. The impulses are initiated in the left ventricle

b. The stimuli are not strong enough to be conducted

c. The ventricle can receive only 120 stimuli in 1 min

d. The AV junction is unable to conduct all the excitation impulses

44. Identify the normal impulse flow of the heart's electrical conduction system:

    1. SA node

    2. Purkinje fibers

    3. Bundle of His

    4. AV node

    5. Bundle branches

    6. Internodal pathways

    a. 1, 5, 2, 4, 6, 3

    b. 1, 6, 4, 3, 5, 2

    c. 1, 4, 3, 6, 5, 2

    d. 1, 2, 3, 4, 5, 6

45. When the EKG shows there is no relationship between the P wave and the QRS complex, you should suspect:

    a. First-degree block

    b. Second-degree block

    c. Third-degree block

    d. Electromechanical dissociation

46. A 65-year-old man presents at the emergency department with severe chest pain. His weight is 75 kg. His heart rate is 40 and his blood pressure (BP) is 70/50. The cardiac monitor shows sinus bradycardia with an occasional premature ventricular complex. Which of the following drugs is indicated first?

    a. Atropine 0.5 mg IV

    b. Isuprel infusion

    c. Lidocaine 75 mg IV bolus

    d. Morphine 10–15 mg IV

47. Administration routes for bretylium include:

    a. IV only

    b. ET only

    c. IO only

    d. IV or ET

48. The pain of stable angina pectoris is:

    a. Predictable

    b. Not predictable

    c. Never very severe

    d. Usually undetectable

49. Signs and symptoms that may be observed in a patient with necrotic heart tissue could include:

a. Dysrhythmias

b. Congestive heart failure

c. Cardiogenic shock (severe)

d. All of the above are possible

50. The term *supraventricular* indicates a stimulus arising above the ventricles.

a. True

b. False

51. The Wenckebach phenomenon differs from complete heart block in that complete heart block has:

a. A faster rate

b. A normal QRS

c. A constant PR Interval

d. A regular RR interval

52. Paroxysmal atrial tachycardia (PAT) is a sudden onset of atrial tachycardia.

a. True

b. False

53. The T wave on the EKG strip represents:

a. Rest period

b. Bundle of His

c. Atrial contraction

d. Ventricular contraction

54. The coronary circulation has how many **main** arteries?

a. 2

b. 6

c. 4

d. 8

55. Starling's law may be expressed as follows:

a. An increase in systolic filling does not alter cardiac output

b. A decrease in systolic filling decreases the force of contraction

c. An increase in diastolic filling increases the force of contraction

d. An increase in filling time yields greater cardiac output regardless of peripheral resistance

56. Inferior wall infarctions are associated with the:

a. Right coronary artery

b. Left coronary artery

c. Bundle of His

d. Coronary sinus

57. Myocardial infarctions may be classified as either transmural or:
    a. Supraendocardial
    b. Subendocardial
    c. Endocardial
    d. Precardial

58. Subendocardial infarctions are commonly referred to as:
    a. Full-thickness
    b. Transmural
    c. Nontransmural
    d. Transdermal

59. Pulseless electrical activity (PEA) may be manifested by:
    a. Normal EKG, normal pulse
    b. Normal or abnormal EKG, absent pulse
    c. Abnormal EKG, normal pulse
    d. Normal or abnormal EKG, absent BP

60. The function of the chordae tendineae and papillary muscles is to:
    a. Prevent backflow of blood into the ventricles
    b. Protect the coronary orifices when the aortic valve opens
    c. Prevent backflow of blood into the atrium
    d. Facilitate backflow of blood from the aorta

61. A 50-year-old man is complaining of chest pain that began while he was clearing underbrush on a vacant lot. He describes the pain as a "heavy pressure" that has lasted 5 to 10 minutes. Vital signs are: BP 140/95, heart rate (HR) 82, respirations 16. The patient has no previous cardiac history. EKG shows normal sinus rhythm. The chest pain is most probably due to:
    a. Dysrhythmias
    b. Pulmonary embolus
    c. Coronary insufficiency
    d. Congestive heart failure

62. Lead II is the lead most commonly used in the prehospital arena because Lead II:
    a. Is the easiest to apply
    b. Shows good T waves
    c. Illustrates good P waves
    d. Is the fastest to apply

63. The ability of certain cardiac cells to initiate excitation impulses spontaneously is called:
    a. Automaticity
    b. Contractility

c. Conductivity

d. Excitability

64. The keys to interpretation of second-degree heart block, Mobitz Type II, are the presence of constant PR Intervals and the fact that there are more P waves present than QRS complexes.

a. True

b. False

65. The absence of electrical impulses results in the recording of a flat line on an EKG strip.

a. False

b. True

66. Your patient is a race car driver who was in a head-on automobile collision. Upon assessment, you immediately notice that the patient has multiple contusions on the chest area. You realize you are probably dealing with:

a. Angina pectoris

b. Myocardial infarction

c. Myocardial trauma

d. Hypertensive crisis

67. A patient complains of substernal chest pain radiating to his left arm and jaw. He has vomited once and still feels nauseated. He is sitting up, appears to be short of breath, and is sweating profusely. Your patient's symptoms most probably are related to:

a. Pacemaker failure

b. Pulmonary edema

c. Hypertensive crisis

d. Acute myocardial infarction

68. If a known coronary bypass patient suffers a cardiac arrest, the health care provider should:

a. Not perform cardiopulmonary resuscitation (CPR) due to the risk of further injury

b. Deliver lighter compressions due to the risk of further injury

c. Provide CPR in the same manner as you would do for any other patient in arrest

d. Provide CPR unless fracture of the sternum or ribs becomes apparent

69. The expected rate of a junctional escape rhythm is:

a. 20–40 BPM

b. 60–100 BPM

c. 40–60 BPM

d. 60–80 BPM

70. When interpreting dysrhythmias, you should remember that the most important key is the:
    a. PR Interval
    b. Rate and rhythm
    c. Presence of dysrhythmias
    d. Patient's clinical appearance

71. In order to obtain a 2-lead EKG strip, you should apply _____ leads to the patient's chest.
    a. 3
    b. 4
    c. 5
    d. 6

72. The uppermost portion of the heart is known as the:
    a. Apex
    b. Base
    c. Atria
    d. Aorta

73. The most common causes of poor EKG tracings are:
    a. Patient movement
    b. Loose leads/electrodes
    c. Both a and b
    d. None of the above

74. "A graphic record of the electrical activity of the heart" describes a(n):
    a. Echocardiogram
    b. Electrocardiogram
    c. Encephalogram
    d. Radiogram

75. The initial treatment for multifocal PVCs should be:
    a. Defibrillation
    b. Cardioversion
    c. Oxygen administration
    d. Pulse oximetry

76. All of the following statements regarding verapamil are correct except:
    a. It may be used to treat paroxysmal supraventricular tachycardia
    b. It causes peripheral vasodilation
    c. It is contraindicated in hypotensive patients
    d. It is indicated in patients with a history of Wolff-Parkinson-White syndrome

77. Atropine is indicated for all the following situations except:

    a. Asystole

    b. Symptomatic third-degree block

    c. Asymptomatic first-degree block

    d. Symptomatic bradycardia

78. In cardiac arrest, Atropine is administered in doses of:

    a. 1.0 mg every 5 min, not to exceed 2 mg

    b. 0.5 mg every 5 min, not to exceed 3 mg

    c. 1.0 mg every 5 min, not to exceed 5 mg

    d. 0.5 mg every 10 min, not to exceed 3 mg

79. The initial bolus of lidocaine should be:

    a. Administered via IV infusion if the patient is complaining of chest pain

    b. Reduced by half if the patient is 70 years old or older

    c. Doubled if the patient is in cardiopulmonary arrest

    d. Titrated to effect if the patient is symptomatic

80. Lidocaine is indicated in all of the following situations except:

    a. Atrial fibrillation with a ventricular rate of 100 BPM

    b. Malignant premature ventricular contractions

    c. Ventricular tachycardia (with palpable pulse)

    d. Symptomatic multifocal premature ventricular contractions

81. Which of the following medications decreases automaticity of the heart?

    a. Isoproterenol

    b. Atropine

    c. Lidocaine

    d. Naloxone

82. A patient may experience side effects of blurred vision, dilated pupils, dry mouth, and flushing of the skin when which drug is administered?

    a. Adenosine

    b. Bretylium

    c. Atropine

    d. Morphine

83. In order for heart rate to be accurately calculated by the R-to-R interval method, the patient must have a regular rhythm.

    a. True

    b. False

84. Second-degree heart block, Type I may be transient and self-correcting.
   a. True
   b. False

85. Cardiovascular disease is the number one cause of death in the United States.
   a. False
   b. True

86. Prompt, definitive intervention has proven effective in preventing many of these deaths.
   a. True
   b. False

87. The innermost lining of the heart is contiguous with the visceral pericardium and is called the:
   a. Endocardium
   b. Pericardium
   c. Myocardium
   d. Epicardium

88. The right and left atria are separated anatomically by the:
   a. Interatrial septum
   b. Bundle of Kent
   c. Interventricular septum
   d. Endocardial mass

89. The right atrium receives blood from the myocardium via the:
   a. Left marginal branch
   b. Inferior vena cava
   c. Great cardiac vein
   d. Internal carotid artery

90. Two examples of atrioventricular valves are the:
   1. Pulmonic valve
   2. Tricuspid valve
   3. Papillary valve
   4. Bicuspid valve

   a. 1 and 2
   b. 2 and 4
   c. 1 and 3
   d. 3 and 4

91. Deoxygenated blood enters the heart through the:
   1. Coronary sinus
   2. Pulmonary artery

3. Superior vena cava

4. Inferior vena cava

a. 1, 2, and 3

b. 2, 3, and 4

c. 2 and 3 only

d. 1, 3, and 4

92. In EKG strips representing dysrhythmias originating in the AV junction, the P wave, if present, will be inverted or absent.

a. True

b. False

93. The amount of blood ejected by the heart in one cardiac contraction is known as:

a. Preload

b. Afterload

c. Cardiac cycle

d. Stroke volume

94. The pressure in the ventricle at the end of diastole is referred to as:

a. Preload

b. Afterload

c. Cardiac output

d. Autonomic

95. The parasympathetic nervous system is mediated by the 10th cranial nerve, which runs from the brain stem to the rectum. This nerve is called the:

a. Optic nerve

b. Vagus nerve

c. Plexus nerve

d. Ganglia nerve

96. The neurotransmitter for the parasympathetic nervous system is acetylcholine. Release of acetylcholine:

1. Slows the heart rate

2. Increases the heart rate

3. Slows atrioventricular conduction

4. Increases atrioventricular conduction

a. 1 and 3

b. 2 and 3

c. 3 and 4

d. 1 and 4

97. Hyperkalemia refers to an increased level of potassium in the blood and can result in decreased automaticity and conduction.

   a. False

   b. True

98. Cardiac function, both electrical and mechanical, is strongly influenced by electrolyte imbalance.

   a. True

   b. False

99. An EKG strip illustrates a regular rhythm, a heart rate of 70, and QRS complexes that are within normal limits. P waves are variable in configuration across the strip. This rhythm is identified as a:

   a. Wandering atrial pacemaker

   b. First-degree heart block

   c. Third-degree heart block

   d. Second-degree heart block, Mobitz Type I

100. Ventricular irritability in the presence of myocardial infarction is:

   a. A precursor to respiratory involvement

   b. Very dangerous and should be treated

   c. To be expected and not a cause for alarm

   d. Highly unlikely if oxygen is administered

101. Prolonged episodes of supraventricular tachycardia may increase myocardial oxygen demand and may thus increase the need for supplemental oxygen therapy.

   a. False

   b. True

102. A progressing PR Interval until such time as a QRS complex is dropped is considered to be:

   a. Third-degree block

   b. Atrial fibrillation

   c. Second-degree AV block, Mobitz Type I

   d. Second-degree AV block, Mobitz Type II

103. Artifact is defined as EKG waveforms produced from sources outside the heart.

   a. True

   b. False

104. Parasympathetic stimulation controls cardiac action by reducing the heart rate, the speed of impulse through the AV node, and the force of atrial contraction. This response is known as the:

   a. Nodal response

   b. Sinoatrial node

c. Neurotransmitter

d. Vagal response

105. An abnormality in conduction through the ventricles may be identified on the EKG tracing by a(n):

a. Distorted, varying P wave pattern

b. Prolonged PR Interval

c. Wide and bizarre QRS complex

d. Elevated ST segment

106. Lidocaine should be considered for suppressing premature ventricular contractions (PVCs) in acute myocardial infarction in which situation?

a. When PVCs are more frequent than 6 per minute or are multifocal

b. In second- or third-degree heart block

c. In the presence of sinus bradycardia

d. In a patient who is known to be allergic to local anesthetics

107. The faster discharging rate of the AV junction in an accelerated junctional rhythm may be due to:

a. Increased automaticity of the AV junction

b. Blockage of the parasympathetic nervous system response

c. Increased excitation of the internodal pathways

d. Increased excitation of the sinoatrial node

108. Paroxysmal junctional tachycardia is often more appropriately called paroxysmal supraventricular tachycardia, since it may be difficult to distinguish this rhythm from paroxysmal atrial tachycardia due to the rapid rate.

a. True

b. False

109. Defibrillation is the treatment of choice for:

1. Asystole

2. Pulseless ventricular tachycardia

3. Ventricular fibrillation

4. Idioventricular rhythms

a. 1, 2, and 3

b. 2 and 3

c. 1, 3, and 4

d. 3 and 4

110. Since unifocal PVCs imply uniform irritability of the entire myocardium, they are generally considered more life-threatening than multifocal PVCs.

a. True

b. False

111. A 69-year-old male is experiencing mild chest pain. Physical exam reveals no other significant findings. Vital signs are: BP 160/88, pulse 84 and irregular, respirations 24. Cardiac monitor reveals a normal sinus rhythm with five unifocal PVCs per minute. The most appropriate treatment is:

a. Monitor patient only, as no treatment is indicated

b. Oxygen via nonrebreathing mask; IV; cardiac monitor

c. Oxygen at 6 l per nasal cannula; IV with D5W/normal saline at keep vein open (KVO) rate; cardiac monitor

d. Oxygen at 10 l per ET tube; rapid IV infusion of lactated Ringer solution; cardiac monitor

112. Which of the following IS NOT a trait of malignant or dangerous PVCs:

a. Unifocal premature complexes

b. R-on-T phenomenon

c. Rate of greater than 6 per minute

d. Runs of ventricular tachycardia

113. All of the following are treatments for ventricular fibrillation:

1. Defibrillate at 200–300 joules

2. Intubate

3. Defibrillate at 200 joules

4. Begin CPR

5. Defibrillate at 360 joules

6. Establish IV access

The correct sequence for these treatments is:

a. 4, 3, 1, 5, 2, 6

b. 4, 2, 5, 1, 3, 6

c. 4, 2, 3, 1, 5, 6

d. 3, 1, 5, 4, 2, 6

114. Your patient is an 82-year-old woman with a history of coronary artery disease. She is conscious and alert. She is complaining of substernal chest pain, radiating to the left arm. She is diaphoretic and short of breath. BP is 120/64, pulse is 56 and irregular, and respirations are 32, shallow, and congested. You connect the cardiac monitor and it shows ventricular fibrillation. Your immediate action is to:

a. Begin CPR

b. Prepare to defibrillate at 200 joules

c. Check the monitor leads

d. Defibrillate at 200 joules

115. Since pacemakers are prone to damage from strong electrical stimuli, you should never defibrillate a patient who has an implanted pacemaker at a setting over 300 joules.

    a. True

    b. False

116. Second-degree AV block (Mobitz Type II) is usually associated with acute myocardial infarction and septal necrosis and is considered to be more serious than the Wenckebach phenomenon.

    a. True

    b. False

117. The point at which the QRS complex meets the ST segment is known as the:

    a. Delta wave

    b. End point

    c. J point

    d. Vector

118. How many cardiac monitor pads are utilized when obtaining a 12-lead EKG?

    a. 10

    b. 12

    c. 3

    d. 6

119. The 12-lead electrocardiogram is used to evaluate all of the following except:

    a. Pulse rate

    b. Valvular dysfunction

    c. Electrical activity in the heart

    d. Isolated waveforms indicative of acute MI (AMI)

120. The right and left coronary arteries branch off of the:

    a. Ventricular artery

    b. Myocardial fossa

    c. Proximal portion of the aorta

    d. Distal portion of the aorta

121. Collateral circulation allows for:

    a. Alternate path of blood flow in the event of occlusion

    b. Circulation continuum during diastole

    c. Maintaining artery patency during spasms

    d. Blood flow continuum during systole

122. Myocardial infarction is:

    a. Always temporary

    b. Not treatable

    c. Age limited in most patients

    d. Due to myocardial cell necrosis

123. The most common cause of the majority of AMIs is:

    a. Coronary vasospasms

    b. Atherosclerotic lesions

    c. Thrombus formation

    d. Arteriosclerotic blebs

124. In acute myocardial infarctions, chest pain is:

    a. Short in duration and relieved by nitroglycerin

    b. Short in duration but not relieved by nitroglycerin

    c. Long in duration and relieved by nitroglycerin

    d. Long in duration and not relieved by nitroglycerin

125. The primary goal of management of the patient with symptomatic chest pain is to:

    a. Interrupt the infarction process

    b. Enhance the infarction process

    c. Institute thrombolytic therapy

    d. Increase myocardial oxygen consumption

126. Management of a patient who is suspected of having sustained a myocardial contusion should:

    a. Focus primarily on the associated and isolated chest injury

    b. Be similar to the treatment administered to a suspected MI patient

    c. Only be initiated at the definitive care facility following transport

    d. Completed in the prehospital arena, prior to transport to the hospital

127. Signs and symptoms the health care provider may expect to observe in a patient with necrotic heart tissue could include:

    a. Dysrhythmias

    b. Congestive heart failure

    c. Cardiogenic shock (severe)

    d. All of the above are possible

128. The right atrium receives blood from the myocardium via the:

    a. Left marginal branch

    b. Inferior vena cava

    c. Great cardiac vein

    d. Internal carotid artery

129. ST segment depression may be evident on a 12-lead EKG strip following both angina and strenuous exercise.

   a. False

   b. True

130. EKG changes of significance with myocardial ischemia include ST segment depression, T wave inversion, or:

   a. Depressed T wave

   b. Peaked T wave

   c. Peaked P wave

   d. Inverted P wave

131. Chest pain should be considered to be cardiac in origin and managed accordingly until proven otherwise.

   a. True

   b. False

132. Leads that record electrical impulses generated from the heart's electrical conduction system and "look at" specific areas of damaged myocardium are called:

   a. Reciprocal leads

   b. Facing leads

   c. Viewing leads

   d. Specific leads

133. The most important diagnostic tool that you can utilize when assessing and treating a patient with a suspected inferior MI is the:

   a. 12-lead EKG machine

   b. Cardiac enzymes

   c. Patient's clinical appearance

   d. Patient's presenting vital signs

134. If ST segment elevation is noted in the lower limb leads (Leads II, III, and aVF), this finding is indicative of:

   a. Anterior myocardial infarction

   b. Lateral myocardial infarction

   c. Superior myocardial infarction

   d. Inferior myocardial infarction

135. If your patient is hypotensive and is exhibiting EKG changes consistent with an inferior myocardial infarction, you should consider the possibility of:

   a. Right atrial infarction

   b. Left atrial infarction

   c. Right ventricular infarction

   d. Left ventricular infarction

136. Any patient who complains of chest pain must be thoroughly evaluated and management should continue until the possibility of AMI is ruled out by the physician.

    a. True

    b. False

137. In the 2-lead method of axis determination, a normal axis is determined by:

    a. Negative QRS deflection in Leads I and aVF

    b. Positive QRS deflection in Leads I and aVF

    c. Negative QRS deflection in Lead I and positive QRS deflection in aVF

    d. Negative QRS deflection in Lead I and positive QRS deflection in aVL

138. In the 2-lead method of axis determination, a left axis deviation is determined by:

    a. Negative QRS deflection in Leads I and aVF

    b. Positive QRS deflection in Leads I and aVF

    c. Negative QRS deflection in Lead I and positive QRS deflection in aVF

    d. Positive QRS deflection in Lead I and negative QRS deflection in aVF

139. In the 2-lead method of axis determination, a right axis deviation is determined by:

    a. Negative QRS deflection in Leads I and aVF

    b. Positive QRS deflection in Leads I and aVF

    c. Negative QRS deflection in Lead I and positive QRS deflection in aVF

    d. Positive QRS deflection in Lead I and negative QRS deflection in aVF

140. In the 2-lead method of axis determination, an indeterminate right axis deviation is determined by:

    a. Negative QRS deflection in Leads I and aVF

    b. Positive QRS deflection in Leads I and aVF

    c. Negative QRS deflection in Lead I and positive QRS deflection in aVF

    d. Positive QRS deflection in Lead I and negative QRS deflection in aVF

141. Which of the following disease processes can be expected in left axis deviation?

    a. Left bundle branch block

    b. Pulmonary hypertension

c. Wolff-Parkinson-White syndrome

d. Ischemic heart disease

142. Which of the following disease processes can be expected in right axis deviation?

   a. Ischemic heart disease

   b. Chronic obstructive pulmonary disease

   c. Right bundle branch block

   d. Systemic hypertension

143. The right bundle branch runs down the right side of the interventricular septum and terminates at the _____ _____ in the right ventricle.

   a. Purkinje network

   b. Papillary muscles

   c. Anterior fascicle

   d. Posterior fascicle

144. To determine right bundle branch block, the primary EKG leads to observe are:

   a. V_1, V_2

   b. V_5, V_6

   c. V_2, V_3

   d. V_2, V_4

145. If ST segment elevation is noted in Leads V_5 and V_6, this finding is indicative of:

   a. Anterior myocardial infarction

   b. Lateral myocardial infarction

   c. Superior myocardial infarction

   d. Inferior myocardial infarction

146. If ST segment depression is noted in V_1, V_2, V_3, and possibly V_4, this finding is indicative of:

   a. Anterior myocardial infarction

   b. Lateral myocardial infarction

   c. Posterior myocardial infarction

   d. Inferior myocardial infarction

147. The combination of posterior wall injury evidence, in addition to evidence of _____, indicates a more extensive infarction and a greater risk of complications.

   a. Anterior wall ischemia

   b. Inferior infarction

   c. T wave inversion

   d. Prolonged PR Interval

148. If ST segment elevation is noted in Leads V_1 and V_2, this finding is indicative of:

a. Anterior myocardial infarction

b. Septal myocardial infarction

c. Superior myocardial infarction

d. Inferior myocardial infarction

149. If ST segment elevation is noted in Leads V_3 and V_4, this finding is indicative of:

a. Anterior myocardial infarction

b. Septal myocardial infarction

c. Superior myocardial infarction

d. Inferior myocardial infarction

150. The drug most commonly used in the treatment of symptomatic bradycardia is:

a. Amiodarone

b. Adenosine

c. Atropine

d. Adrenalin

18

12-LEAD EKG
REVIEW STRIPS

The review strips in this chapter are presented to enhance your ability to interpret 12-Lead EKGs. Although the answers are provided in Appendix 2, we strongly encourage you to apply the 5 + 3 approach to each review strip *before* you refer to the answer. We trust that this chapter will prove valuable to you. Good luck!

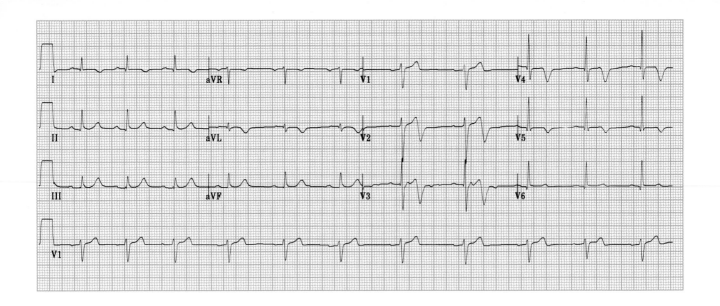

1

1. Rate: _____ 2. Rhythm: _____ 3. P wave: _____

4. PR Interval: _____ 5. QRS complex: _____ +1. ST elevation: _____

+2. ST depression: _____ +3. Pathologic Q waves: _____ Interpretation: _____

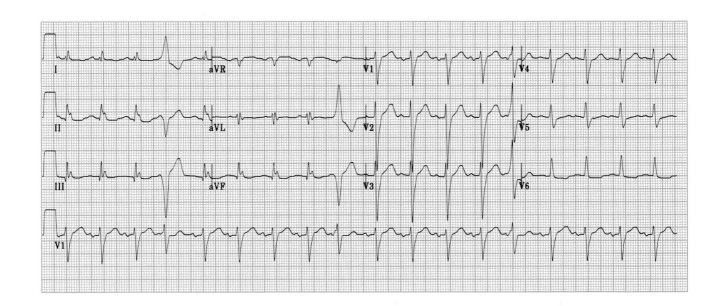

2

1. Rate: _____ 2. Rhythm: _____ 3. P wave: _____

4. PR Interval: _____ 5. QRS complex: _____ +1. ST elevation: _____

+2. ST depression: _____ +3. Pathologic Q waves: _____ Interpretation: _____

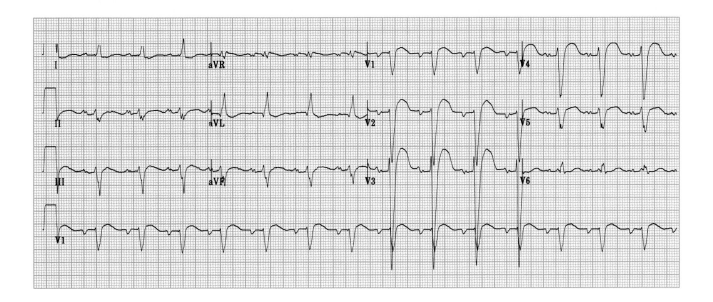

3

1. Rate: _____

2. Rhythm: _____

3. P wave: _____

4. PR Interval: _____

5. QRS complex: _____

+1. ST elevation: _____

+2. ST depression: _____

+3. Pathologic Q waves: _____

Interpretation: _____

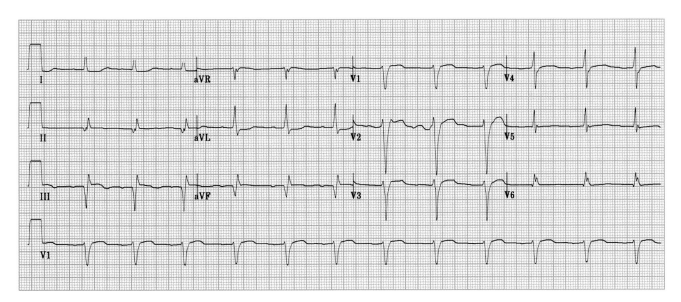

4

1. Rate: _____

2. Rhythm: _____

3. P wave: _____

4. PR Interval: _____

5. QRS complex: _____

+1. ST elevation: _____

+2. ST depression: _____

+3. Pathologic Q waves: _____

Interpretation: _____

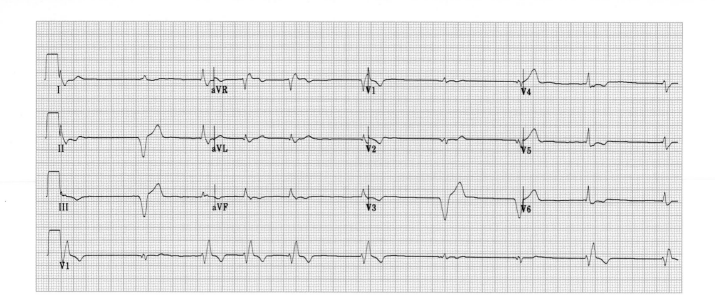

5

1. Rate: _____ 2. Rhythm:_____ 3. P wave: _____

4. PR Interval: _____ 5. QRS complex: _____ +1. ST elevation: _____

+2. ST depression: _____ +3. Pathologic Q waves: _____ Interpretation: _____

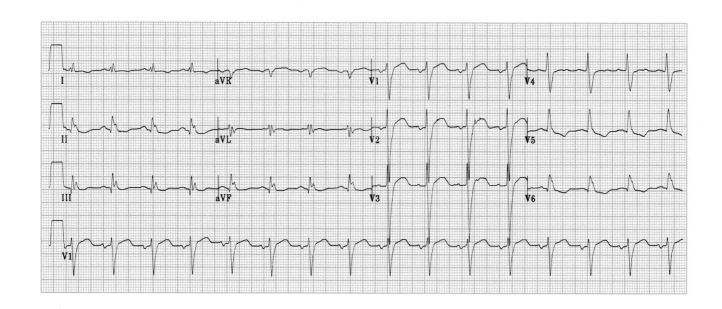

6

1. Rate: _____ 2. Rhythm:_____ 3. P wave: _____

4. PR Interval: _____ 5. QRS complex: _____ +1. ST elevation: _____

+2. ST depression: _____ +3. Pathologic Q waves: _____ Interpretation: _____

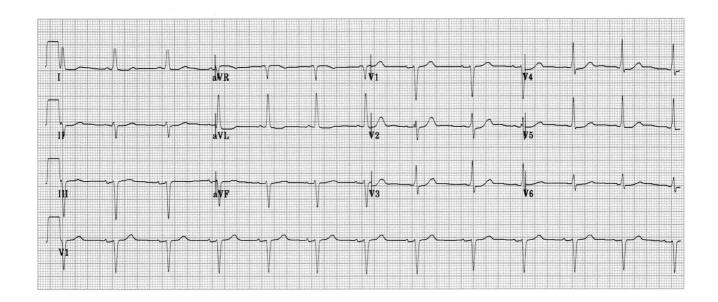

7

1. Rate: _____

2. Rhythm: _____

3. P wave: _____

4. PR Interval: _____

5. QRS complex: _____

+1. ST elevation: _____

+2. ST depression: _____

+3. Pathologic Q waves: _____

Interpretation: _____

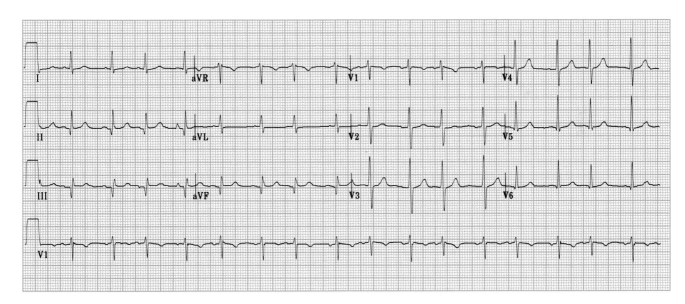

8

1. Rate: _____

2. Rhythm: _____

3. P wave: _____

4. PR Interval: _____

5. QRS complex: _____

+1. ST elevation: _____

+2. ST depression: _____

+3. Pathologic Q waves: _____

Interpretation: _____

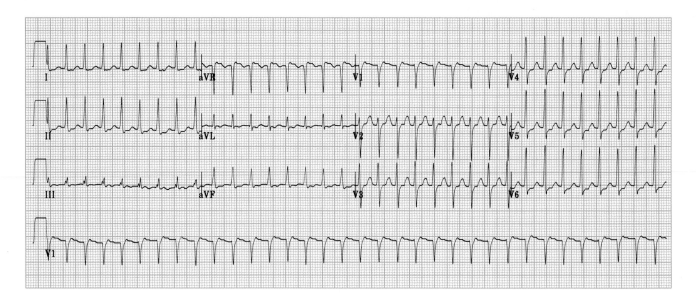

9

1. Rate: _____   2. Rhythm: _____   3. P wave: _____

4. PR Interval: _____   5. QRS complex: _____   +1. ST elevation: _____

+2. ST depression: _____   +3. Pathologic Q waves: _____   Interpretation: _____

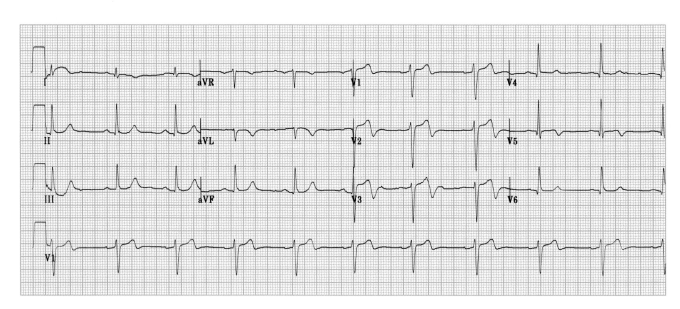

10

1. Rate: _____   2. Rhythm: _____   3. P wave: _____

4. PR Interval: _____   5. QRS complex: _____   +1. ST elevation: _____

+2. ST depression: _____   +3. Pathologic Q waves: _____   Interpretation: _____

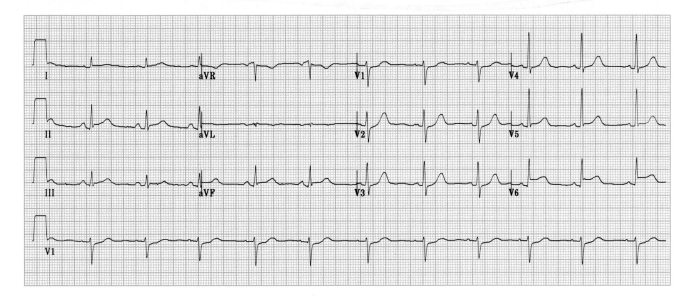

11

1. Rate: _____

2. Rhythm: _____

3. P wave: _____

4. PR Interval: _____

5. QRS complex: _____

+1. ST elevation: _____

+2. ST depression: _____

+3. Pathologic Q waves: _____

Interpretation: _____

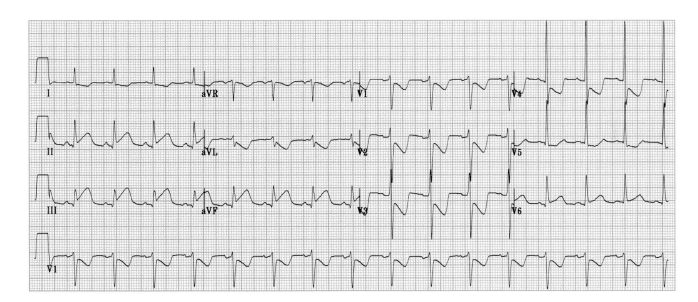

12

1. Rate: _____

2. Rhythm: _____

3. P wave: _____

4. PR Interval: _____

5. QRS complex: _____

+1. ST elevation: _____

+2. ST depression: _____

+3. Pathologic Q waves: _____

Interpretation: _____

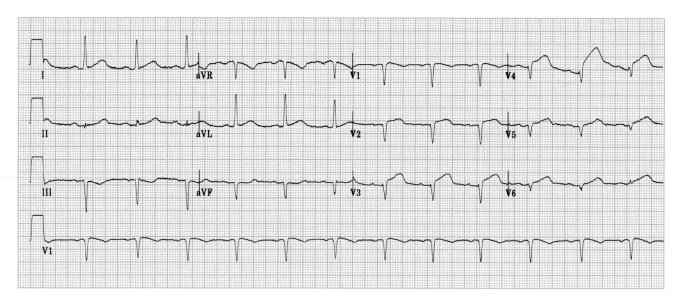

13

1. Rate: _____   2. Rhythm: _____   3. P wave: _____

4. PR Interval: _____   5. QRS complex: _____   +1. ST elevation: _____

+2. ST depression: _____   +3. Pathologic Q waves: _____   Interpretation: _____

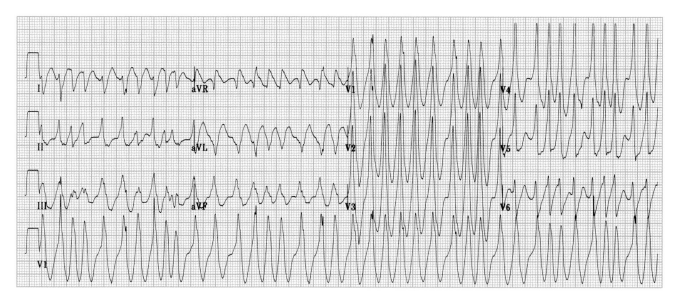

14

1. Rate: _____   2. Rhythm: _____   3. P wave: _____

4. PR Interval: _____   5. QRS complex: _____   +1. ST elevation: _____

+2. ST depression: _____   +3. Pathologic Q waves: _____   Interpretation: _____

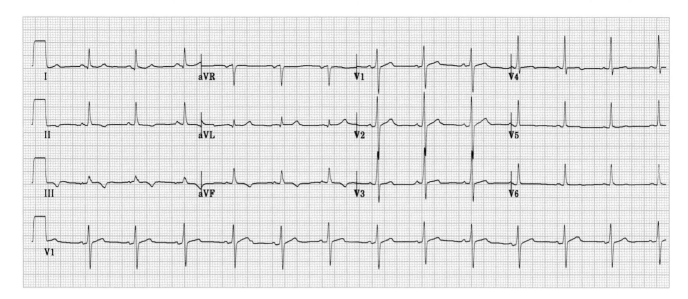

15

1. Rate: _____

2. Rhythm: _____

3. P wave: _____

4. PR Interval: _____

5. QRS complex: _____

+1. ST elevation: _____

+2. ST depression: _____

+3. Pathologic Q waves: _____

Interpretation: _____

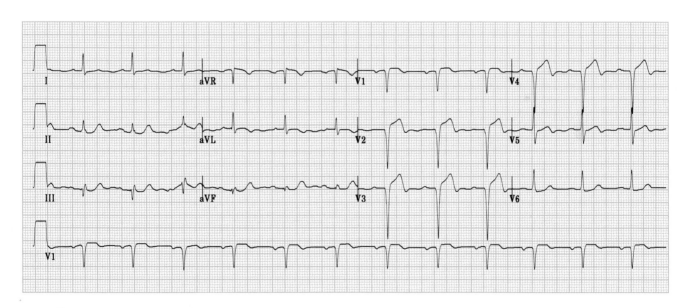

16

1. Rate: _____

2. Rhythm: _____

3. P wave: _____

4. PR Interval: _____

5. QRS complex: _____

+1. ST elevation: _____

+2. ST depression: _____

+3. Pathologic Q waves: _____

Interpretation: _____

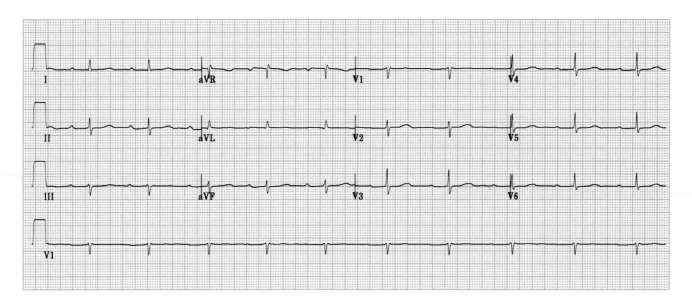

17

1. Rate: _____

2. Rhythm: _____

3. P wave: _____

4. PR Interval: _____

5. QRS complex: _____

+1. ST elevation: _____

+2. ST depression: _____

+3. Pathologic Q waves: _____

Interpretation: _____

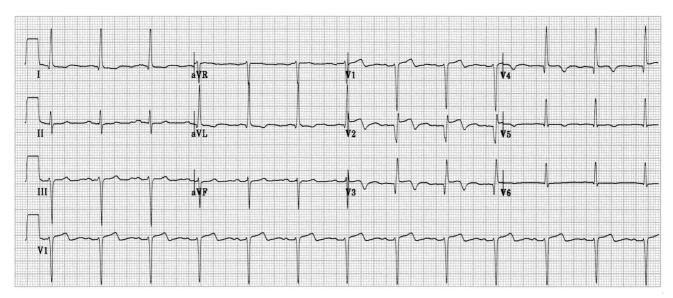

18

1. Rate: _____

2. Rhythm: _____

3. P wave: _____

4. PR Interval: _____

5. QRS complex: _____

+1. ST elevation: _____

+2. ST depression: _____

+3. Pathologic Q waves: _____

Interpretation: _____

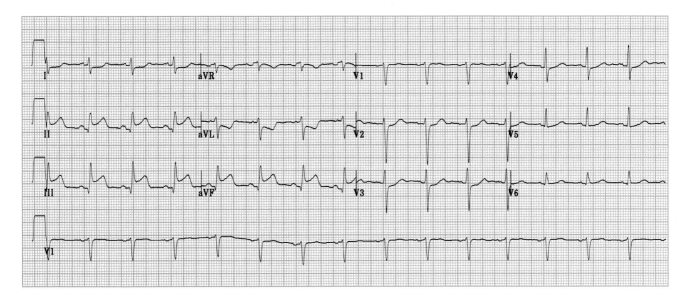

19

1. Rate: _____   2. Rhythm: _____   3. P wave: _____

4. PR Interval: _____   5. QRS complex: _____   +1. ST elevation: _____

+2. ST depression: _____   +3. Pathologic Q waves: _____   Interpretation: _____

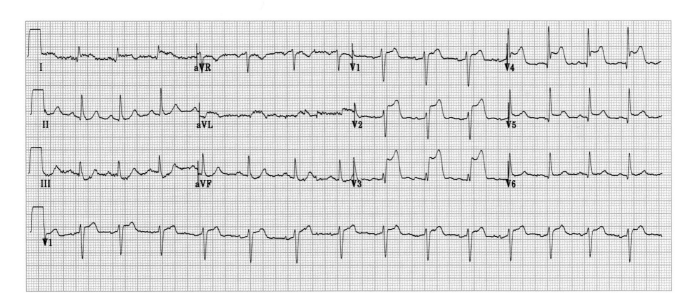

20

1. Rate: _____   2. Rhythm: _____   3. P wave: _____

4. PR Interval: _____   5. QRS complex: _____   +1. ST elevation: _____

+2. ST depression: _____   +3. Pathologic Q waves: _____   Interpretation: _____

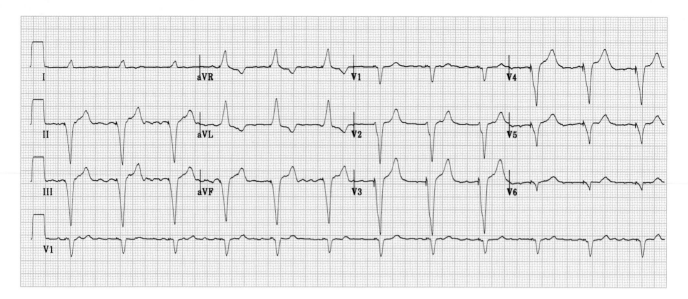

21

1. Rate: _____   2. Rhythm: _____   3. P wave: _____

4. PR Interval: _____   5. QRS complex: _____   +1. ST elevation: _____

+2. ST depression: _____   +3. Pathologic Q waves: _____   Interpretation: _____

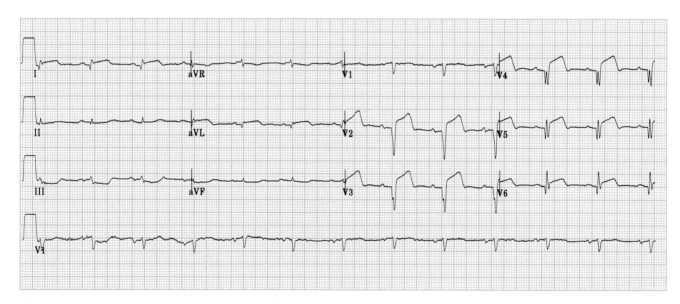

22

1. Rate: _____   2. Rhythm: _____   3. P wave: _____

4. PR Interval: _____   5. QRS complex: _____   +1. ST elevation: _____

+2. ST depression: _____   +3. Pathologic Q waves: _____   Interpretation: _____

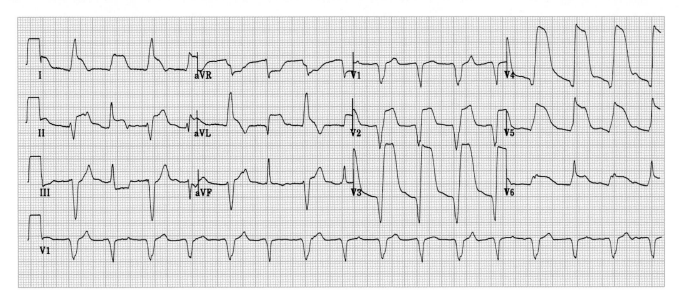

23

1. Rate: _____

2. Rhythm: _____

3. P wave: _____

4. PR Interval: _____

5. QRS complex: _____

+1. ST elevation: _____

+2. ST depression: _____

+3. Pathologic Q waves: _____

Interpretation: _____

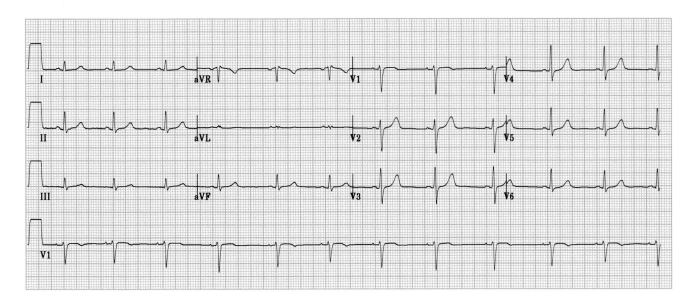

24

1. Rate: _____

2. Rhythm: _____

3. P wave: _____

4. PR Interval: _____

5. QRS complex: _____

+1. ST elevation: _____

+2. ST depression: _____

+3. Pathologic Q waves: _____

Interpretation: _____

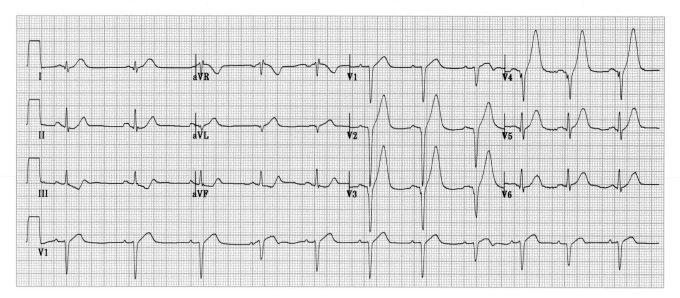

25

1. Rate: _____

2. Rhythm: _____

3. P wave: _____

4. PR Interval: _____

5. QRS complex: _____

+1. ST elevation: _____

+2. ST depression: _____

+3. Pathologic Q waves: _____

Interpretation: _____

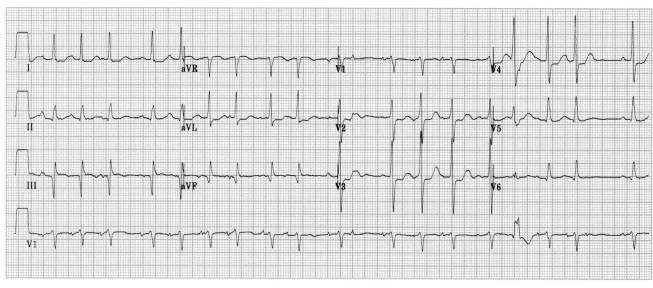

26

1. Rate: _____

2. Rhythm: _____

3. P wave: _____

4. PR Interval: _____

5. QRS complex: _____

+1. ST elevation: _____

+2. ST depression: _____

+3. Pathologic Q waves: _____

Interpretation: _____

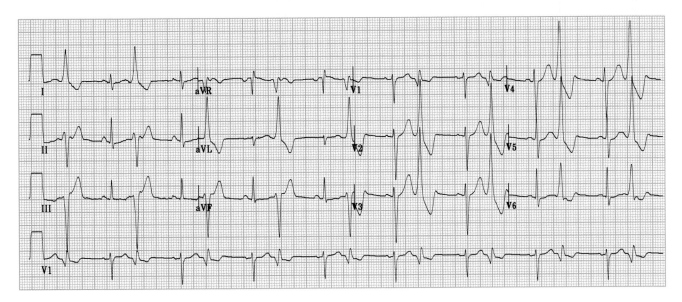

27

1. Rate: _____

2. Rhythm: _____

3. P wave: _____

4. PR Interval: _____

5. QRS complex: _____

+1. ST elevation: _____

+2. ST depression: _____

+3. Pathologic Q waves: _____

Interpretation: _____

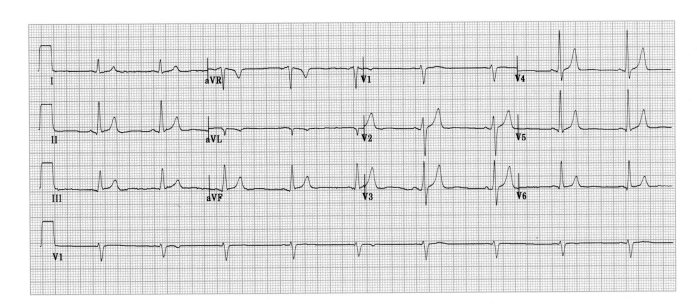

28

1. Rate: _____

2. Rhythm: _____

3. P wave: _____

4. PR Interval: _____

5. QRS complex: _____

+1. ST elevation: _____

+2. ST depression: _____

+3. Pathologic Q waves: _____

Interpretation: _____

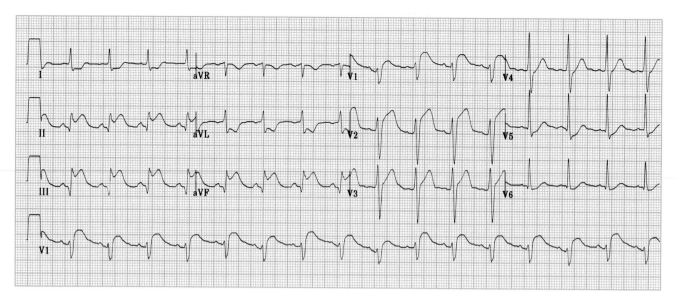

29

1. Rate: _____

2. Rhythm: _____

3. P wave: _____

4. PR Interval: _____

5. QRS complex: _____

+1. ST elevation: _____

+2. ST depression: _____

+3. Pathologic Q waves: _____

Interpretation: _____

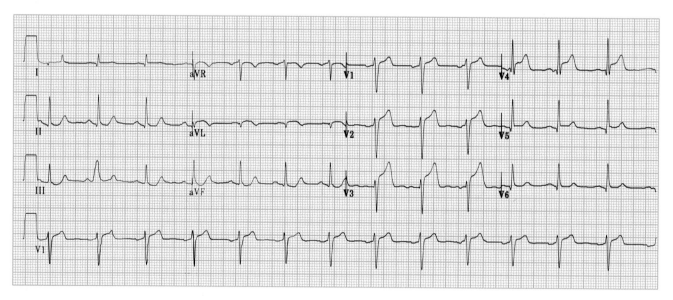

30

1. Rate: _____

2. Rhythm: _____

3. P wave: _____

4. PR Interval: _____

5. QRS complex: _____

+1. ST elevation: _____

+2. ST depression: _____

+3. Pathologic Q waves: _____

Interpretation: _____

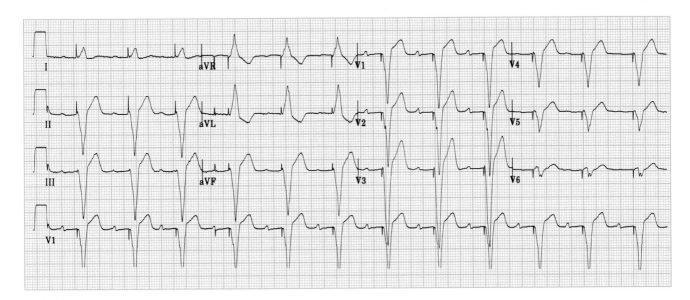

31

1. Rate: _____

2. Rhythm: _____

3. P wave: _____

4. PR Interval: _____

5. QRS complex: _____

+1. ST elevation: _____

+2. ST depression: _____

+3. Pathologic Q waves: _____

Interpretation: _____

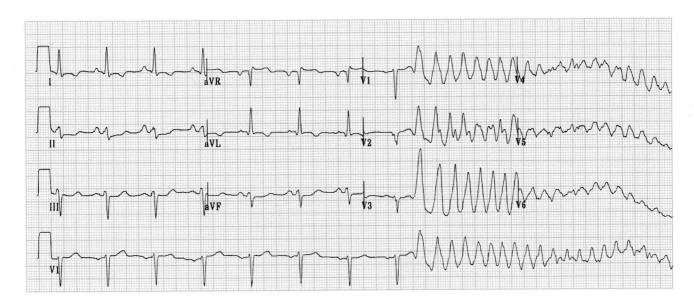

32

1. Rate: _____

2. Rhythm: _____

3. P wave: _____

4. PR Interval: _____

5. QRS complex: _____

+1. ST elevation: _____

+2. ST depression: _____

+3. Pathologic Q waves: _____

Interpretation: _____

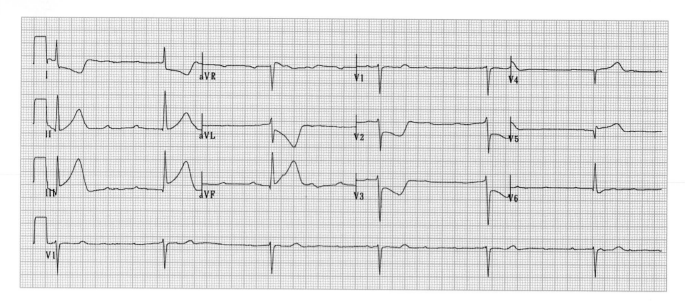

33

1. Rate: _____

2. Rhythm: _____

3. P wave: _____

4. PR Interval: _____

5. QRS complex: _____

+1. ST elevation: _____

+2. ST depression: _____

+3. Pathologic Q waves: _____

Interpretation: _____

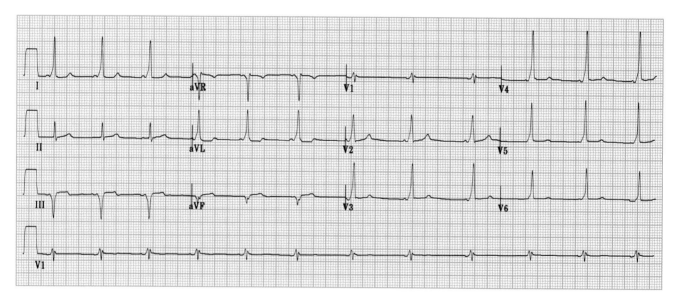

34

1. Rate: _____

2. Rhythm: _____

3. P wave: _____

4. PR Interval: _____

5. QRS complex: _____

+1. ST elevation: _____

+2. ST depression: _____

+3. Pathologic Q waves: _____

Interpretation: _____

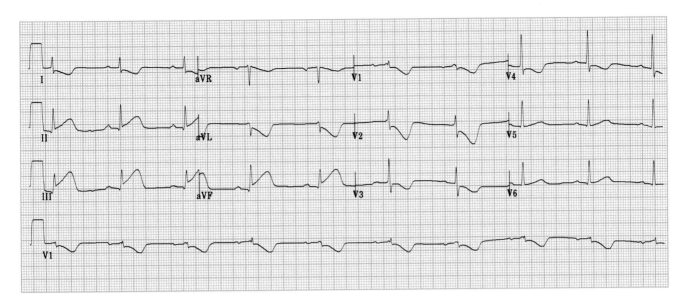

35

1. Rate: _____

4. PR Interval: _____

+2. ST depression: _____

2. Rhythm: _____

5. QRS complex: _____

+3. Pathologic Q waves: _____

3. P wave: _____

+1. ST elevation: _____

Interpretation: _____

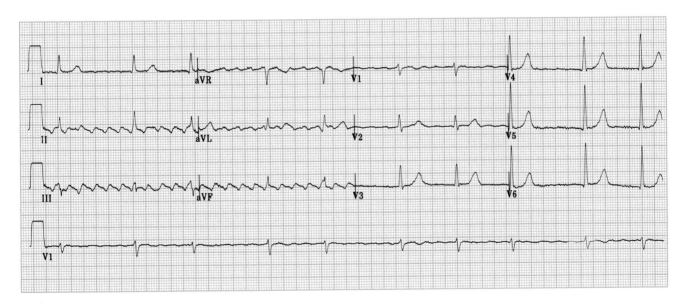

36

1. Rate: _____

4. PR Interval: _____

+2. ST depression: _____

2. Rhythm: _____

5. QRS complex: _____

+3. Pathologic Q waves: _____

3. P wave: _____

+1. ST elevation: _____

Interpretation: _____

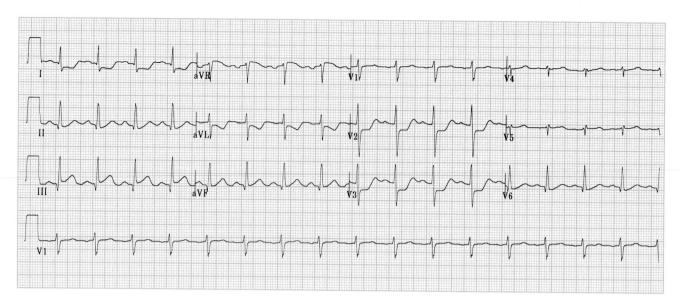

37

1. Rate: _____
2. Rhythm: _____
3. P wave: _____
4. PR Interval: _____
5. QRS complex: _____
+1. ST elevation: _____
+2. ST depression: _____
+3. Pathologic Q waves: _____
Interpretation: _____

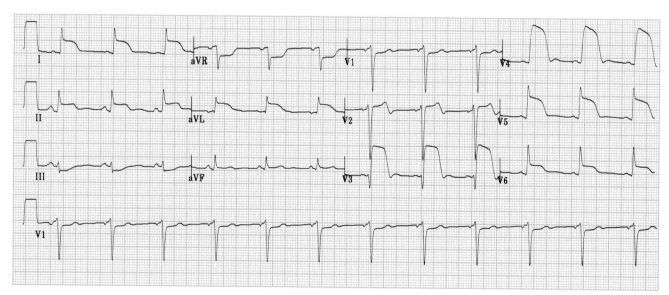

38

1. Rate: _____
2. Rhythm: _____
3. P wave: _____
4. PR Interval: _____
5. QRS complex: _____
+1. ST elevation: _____
+2. ST depression: _____
+3. Pathologic Q waves: _____
Interpretation: _____

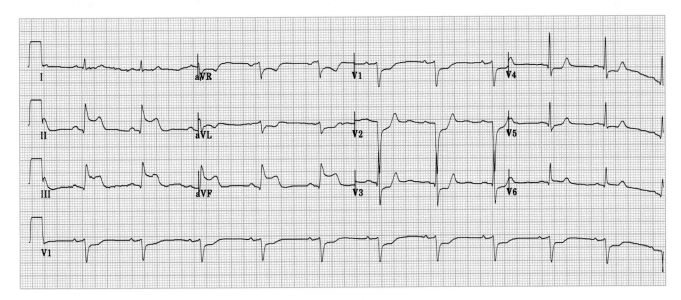

39

1. Rate: _____
2. Rhythm: _____
3. P wave: _____
4. PR Interval: _____
5. QRS complex: _____
+1. ST elevation: _____
+2. ST depression: _____
+3. Pathologic Q waves: _____
Interpretation: _____

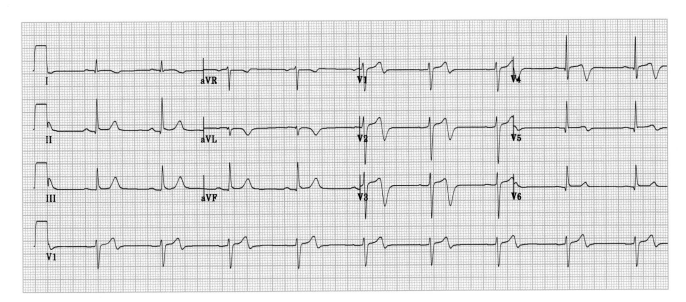

40

1. Rate: _____
2. Rhythm: _____
3. P wave: _____
4. PR Interval: _____
5. QRS complex: _____
+1. ST elevation: _____
+2. ST depression: _____
+3. Pathologic Q waves: _____
Interpretation: _____

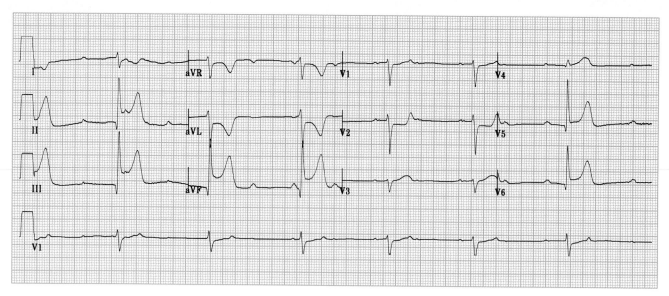

41

1. Rate: _____

2. Rhythm: _____

3. P wave: _____

4. PR Interval: _____

5. QRS complex: _____

+1. ST elevation: _____

+2. ST depression: _____

+3. Pathologic Q waves: _____

Interpretation: _____

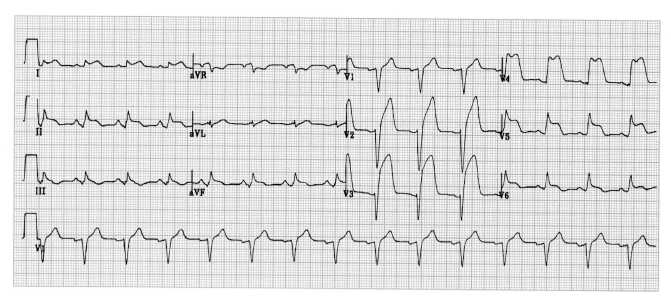

42

1. Rate: _____

2. Rhythm: _____

3. P wave: _____

4. PR Interval: _____

5. QRS complex: _____

+1. ST elevation: _____

+2. ST depression: _____

+3. Pathologic Q waves: _____

Interpretation: _____

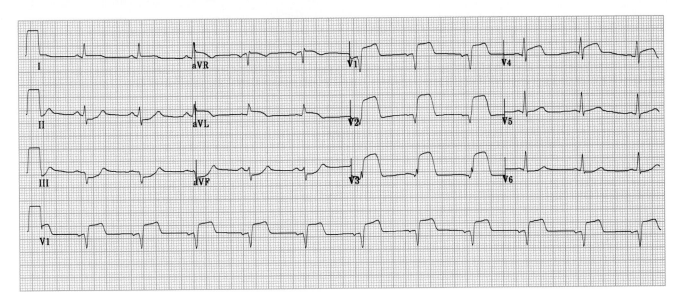

43

1. Rate: _____

4. PR Interval: _____

+2. ST depression: _____

2. Rhythm: _____

5. QRS complex: _____

+3. Pathologic Q waves: _____

3. P wave: _____

+1. ST elevation: _____

Interpretation: _____

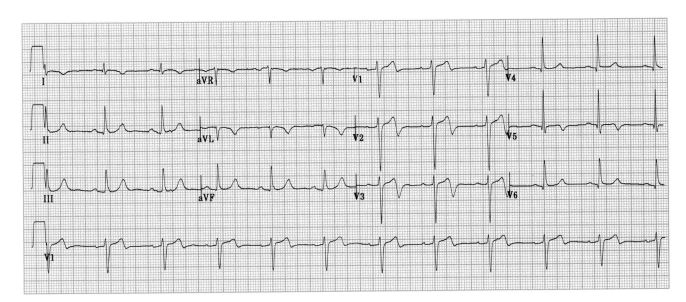

44

1. Rate: _____

4. PR Interval: _____

+2. ST depression: _____

2. Rhythm: _____

5. QRS complex: _____

+3. Pathologic Q waves: _____

3. P wave: _____

+1. ST elevation: _____

Interpretation: _____

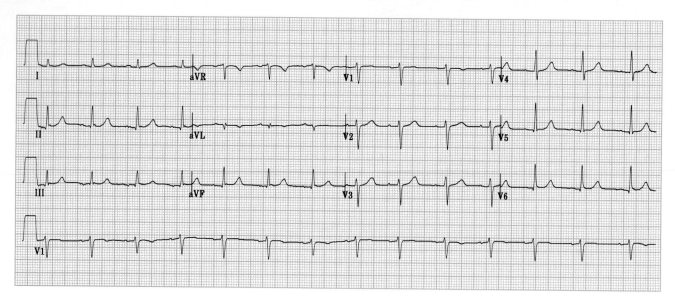

45

1. Rate: _____   2. Rhythm: _____   3. P wave: _____

4. PR Interval: _____   5. QRS complex: _____   +1. ST elevation: _____

+2. ST depression: _____   +3. Pathologic Q waves: _____   Interpretation: _____

46

1. Rate: _____   2. Rhythm: _____   3. P wave: _____

4. PR Interval: _____   5. QRS complex: _____   +1. ST elevation: _____

+2. ST depression: _____   +3. Pathologic Q waves: _____   Interpretation: _____

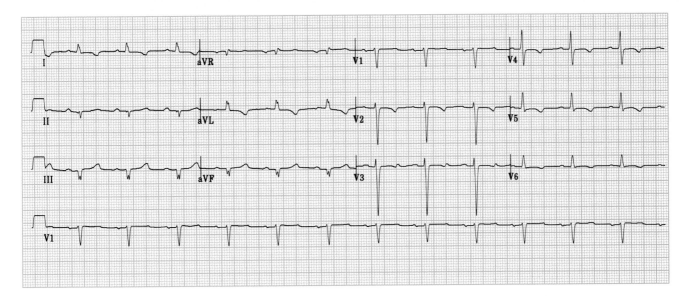

47

1. Rate: _____

2. Rhythm: _____

3. P wave: _____

4. PR Interval: _____

5. QRS complex: _____

+1. ST elevation: _____

+2. ST depression: _____

+3. Pathologic Q waves: _____

Interpretation: _____

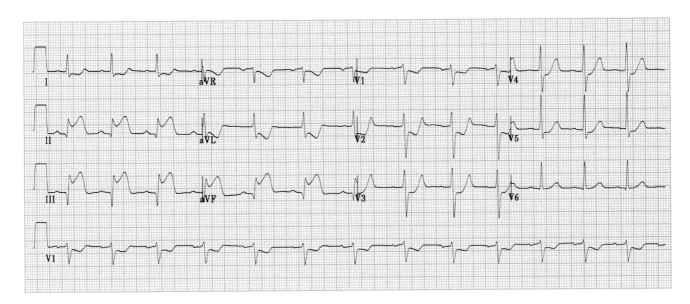

48

1. Rate: _____

2. Rhythm: _____

3. P wave: _____

4. PR Interval: _____

5. QRS complex: _____

+1. ST elevation: _____

+2. ST depression: _____

+3. Pathologic Q waves: _____

Interpretation: _____

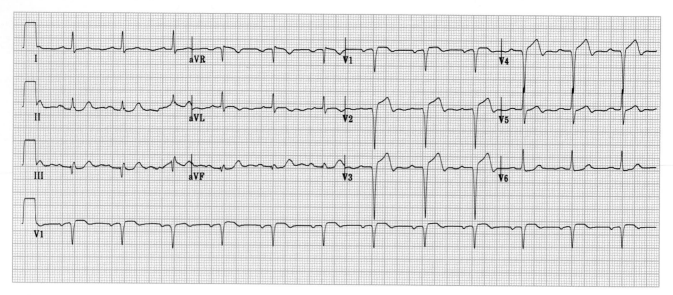

49

1. Rate: _____

2. Rhythm: _____

3. P wave: _____

4. PR Interval: _____

5. QRS complex: _____

+1. ST elevation: _____

+2. ST depression: _____

+3. Pathologic Q waves: _____

Interpretation: _____

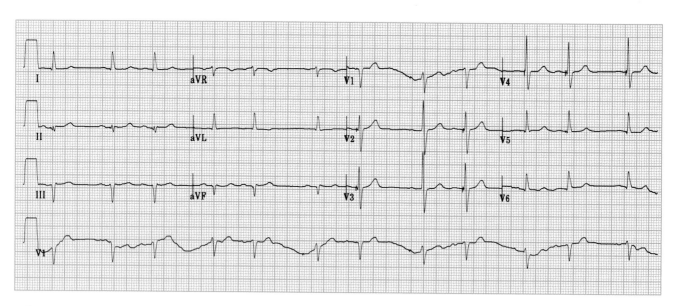

50

1. Rate: _____

2. Rhythm: _____

3. P wave: _____

4. PR Interval: _____

5. QRS complex: _____

+1. ST elevation: _____

+2. ST depression: _____

+3. Pathologic Q waves: _____

Interpretation: _____

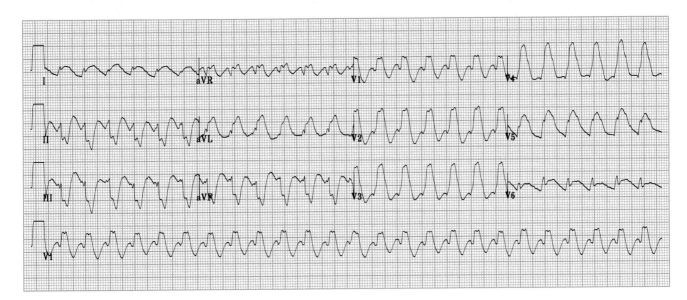

51

1. Rate: _____

4. PR Interval: _____

+2. ST depression: _____

2. Rhythm: _____

5. QRS complex: _____

+3. Pathologic Q waves: _____

3. P wave: _____

+1. ST elevation: _____

Interpretation: _____

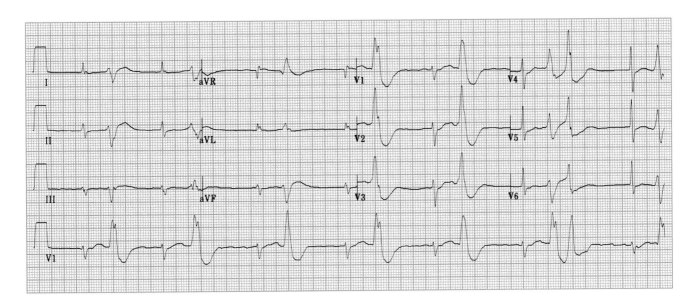

52

1. Rate: _____

4. PR Interval: _____

+2. ST depression: _____

2. Rhythm: _____

5. QRS complex: _____

+3. Pathologic Q waves: _____

3. P wave: _____

+1. ST elevation: _____

Interpretation: _____

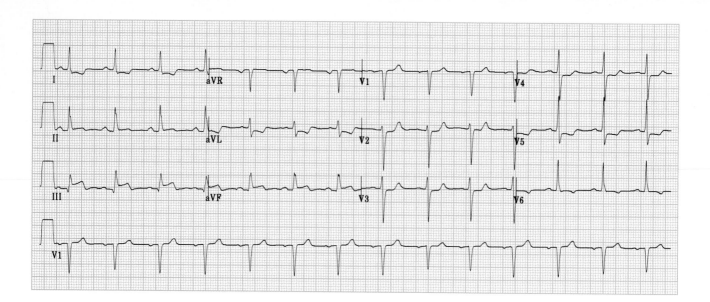

53

1. Rate: _____

2. Rhythm: _____

3. P wave: _____

4. PR Interval: _____

5. QRS complex: _____

+1. ST elevation: _____

+2. ST depression: _____

+3. Pathologic Q waves: _____

Interpretation: _____

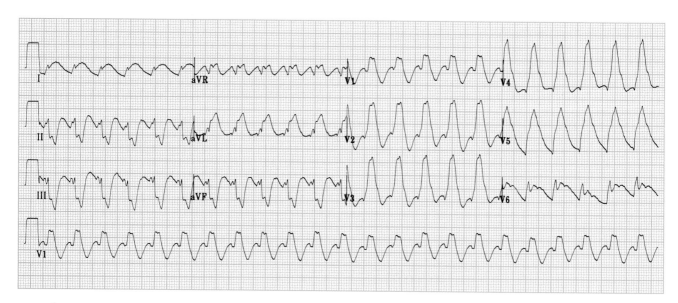

54

1. Rate: _____

2. Rhythm: _____

3. P wave: _____

4. PR Interval: _____

5. QRS complex: _____

+1. ST elevation: _____

+2. ST depression: _____

+3. Pathologic Q waves: _____

Interpretation: _____

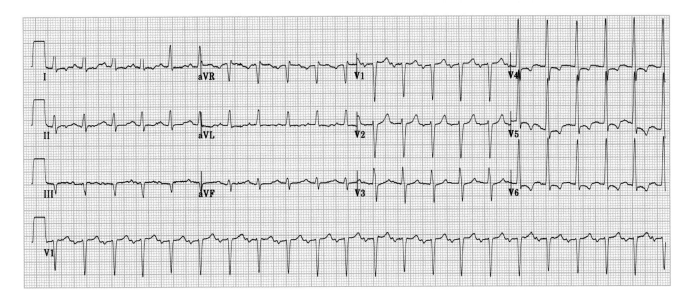

55

1. Rate: _____

4. PR Interval: _____

+2. ST depression: _____

2. Rhythm: _____

5. QRS complex: _____

+3. Pathologic Q waves: _____

3. P wave: _____

+1. ST elevation: _____

Interpretation: _____

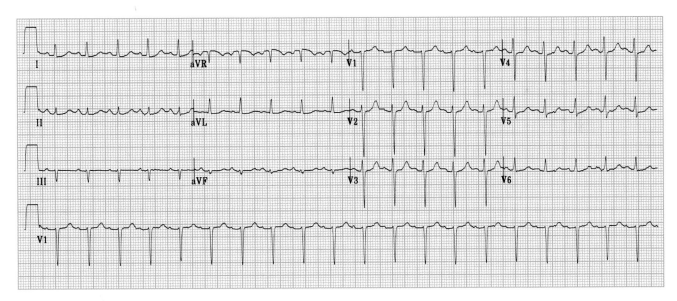

56

1. Rate: _____

4. PR Interval: _____

+2. ST depression: _____

2. Rhythm: _____

5. QRS complex: _____

+3. Pathologic Q waves: _____

3. P wave: _____

+1. ST elevation: _____

Interpretation: _____

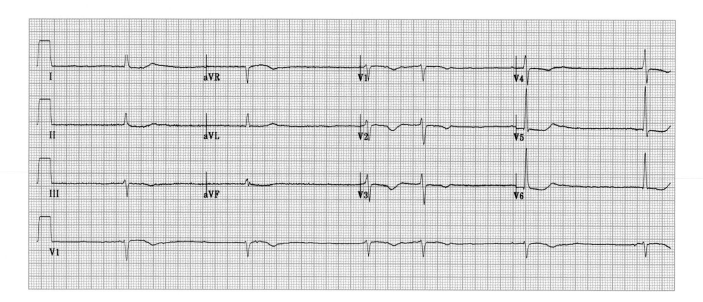

57

1. Rate: _____ 2. Rhythm: _____ 3. P wave: _____

4. PR Interval: _____ 5. QRS complex: _____ +1. ST elevation: _____

+2. ST depression: _____ +3. Pathologic Q waves: _____ Interpretation: _____

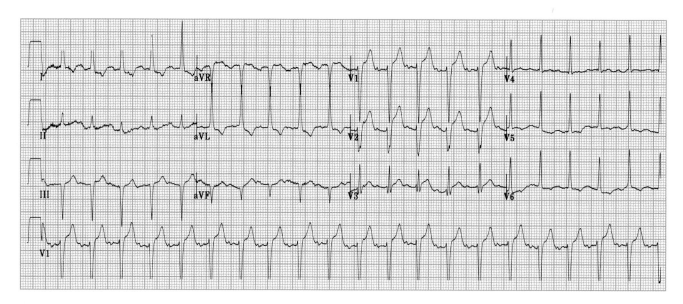

58

1. Rate: _____ 2. Rhythm: _____ 3. P wave: _____

4. PR Interval: _____ 5. QRS complex: _____ +1. ST elevation: _____

+2. ST depression: _____ +3. Pathologic Q waves: _____ Interpretation: _____

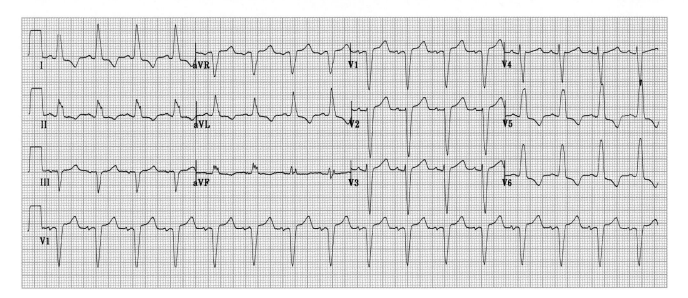

59

1. Rate: _____

2. Rhythm: _____

3. P wave: _____

4. PR Interval: _____

5. QRS complex: _____

+1. ST elevation: _____

+2. ST depression: _____

+3. Pathologic Q waves: _____

Interpretation: _____

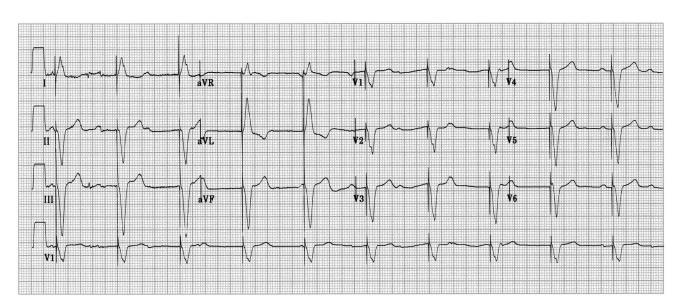

60

1. Rate: _____

2. Rhythm: _____

3. P wave: _____

4. PR Interval: _____

5. QRS complex: _____

+1. ST elevation: _____

+2. ST depression: _____

+3. Pathologic Q waves: _____

Interpretation: _____

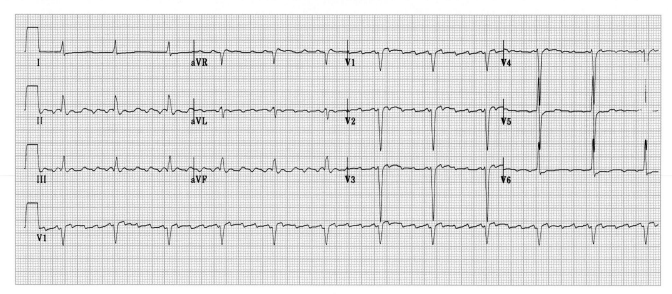

61

1. Rate: _____   2. Rhythm: _____   3. P wave: _____

4. PR Interval: _____   5. QRS complex: _____   +1. ST elevation: _____

+2. ST depression: _____   +3. Pathologic Q waves: _____   Interpretation: _____

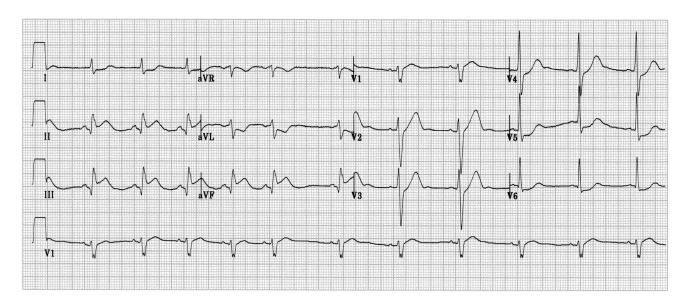

62

1. Rate: _____   2. Rhythm: _____   3. P wave: _____

4. PR Interval: _____   5. QRS complex: _____   +1. ST elevation: _____

+2. ST depression: _____   +3. Pathologic Q waves: _____   Interpretation: _____

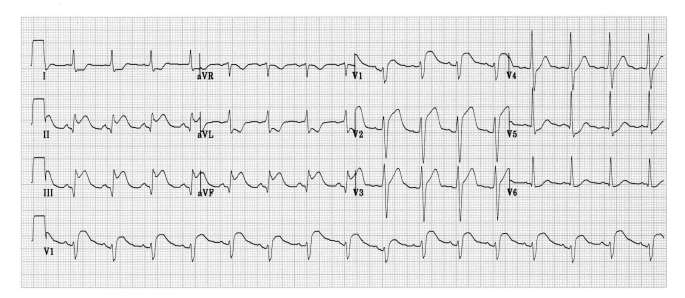

63

1. Rate: _____

2. Rhythm: _____

3. P wave: _____

4. PR Interval: _____

5. QRS complex: _____

+1. ST elevation: _____

+2. ST depression: _____

+3. Pathologic Q waves: _____

Interpretation: _____

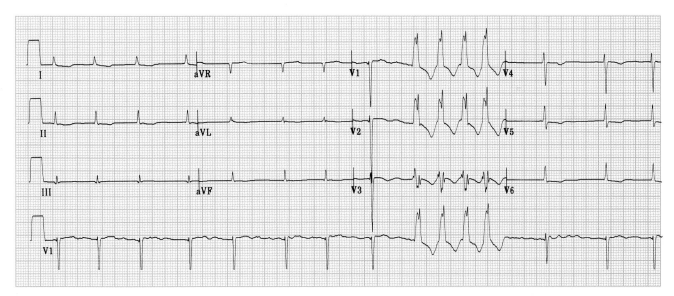

64

1. Rate: _____

2. Rhythm: _____

3. P wave: _____

4. PR Interval: _____

5. QRS complex: _____

+1. ST elevation: _____

+2. ST depression: _____

+3. Pathologic Q waves: _____

Interpretation: _____

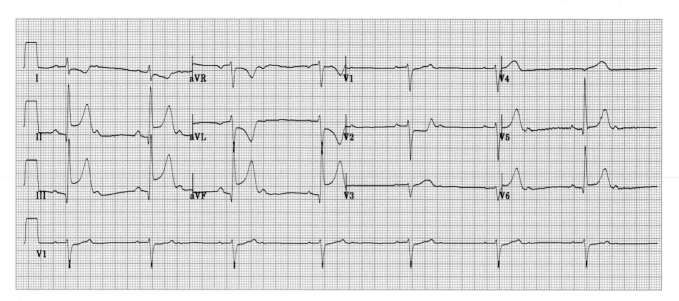

65

1. Rate: _____

2. Rhythm: _____

3. P wave: _____

4. PR Interval: _____

5. QRS complex: _____

+1. ST elevation: _____

+2. ST depression: _____

+3. Pathologic Q waves: _____

Interpretation: _____

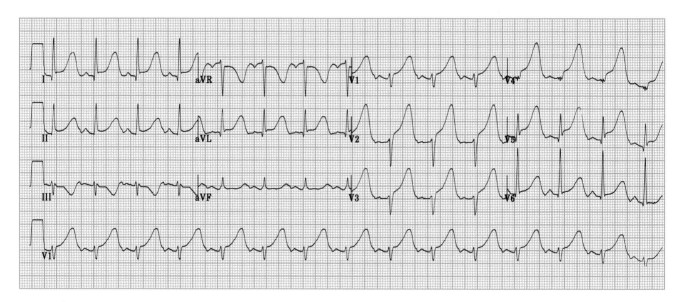

66

1. Rate: _____

2. Rhythm: _____

3. P wave: _____

4. PR Interval: _____

5. QRS complex: _____

+1. ST elevation: _____

+2. ST depression: _____

+3. Pathologic Q waves: _____

Interpretation: _____

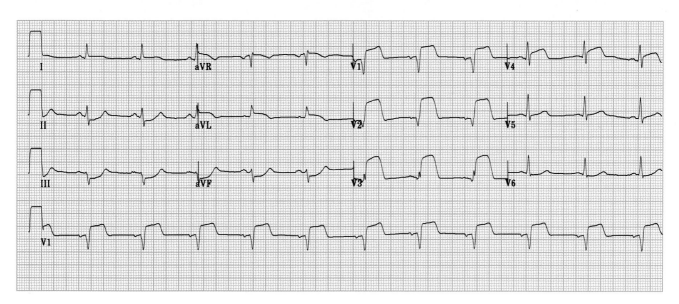

67

1. Rate: _____

2. Rhythm: _____

3. P wave: _____

4. PR Interval: _____

5. QRS complex: _____

+1. ST elevation: _____

+2. ST depression: _____

+3. Pathologic Q waves: _____

Interpretation: _____

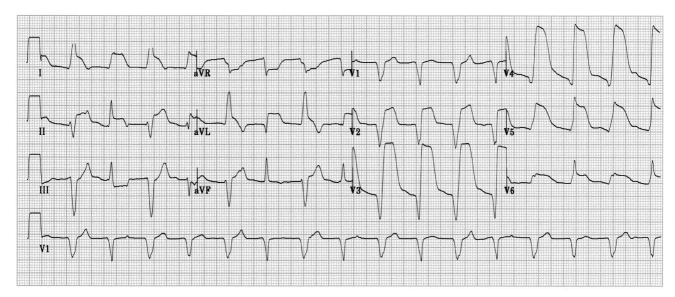

68

1. Rate: _____

2. Rhythm: _____

3. P wave: _____

4. PR Interval: _____

5. QRS complex: _____

+1. ST elevation: _____

+2. ST depression: _____

+3. Pathologic Q waves: _____

Interpretation: _____

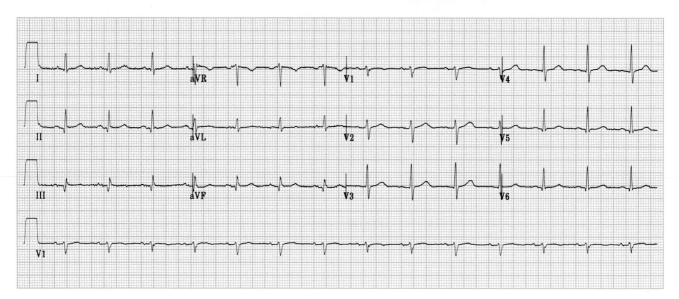

69

1. Rate: _____

4. PR Interval: _____

+2. ST depression: _____

2. Rhythm: _____

5. QRS complex: _____

+3. Pathologic Q waves: _____

3. P wave: _____

+1. ST elevation: _____

Interpretation: _____

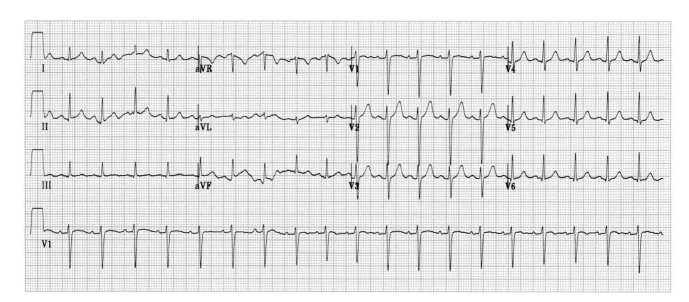

70

1. Rate: _____

4. PR Interval: _____

+2. ST depression: _____

2. Rhythm: _____

5. QRS complex: _____

+3. Pathologic Q waves: _____

3. P wave: _____

+1. ST elevation: _____

Interpretation: _____

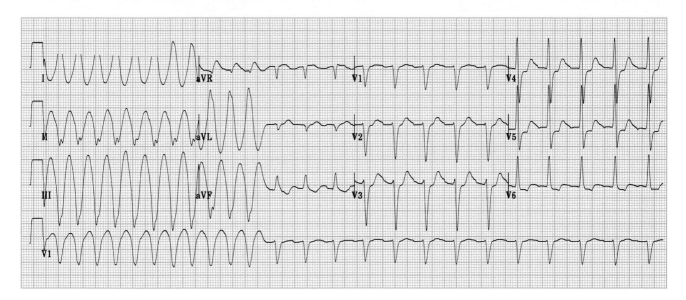

71

1. Rate: _____

2. Rhythm: _____

3. P wave: _____

4. PR Interval: _____

5. QRS complex: _____

+1. ST elevation: _____

+2. ST depression: _____

+3. Pathologic Q waves: _____

Interpretation: _____

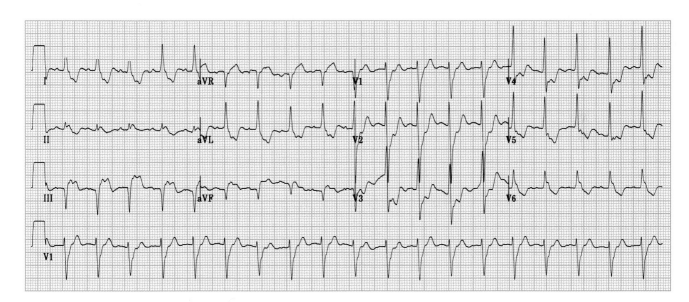

72

1. Rate: _____

2. Rhythm: _____

3. P wave: _____

4. PR Interval: _____

5. QRS complex: _____

+1. ST elevation: _____

+2. ST depression: _____

+3. Pathologic Q waves: _____

Interpretation: _____

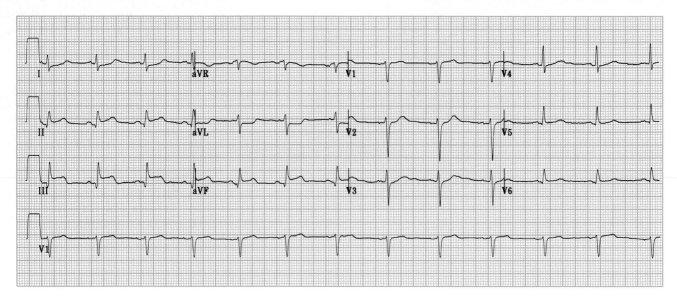

73

1. Rate: _____ 2. Rhythm: _____ 3. P wave: _____

4. PR Interval: _____ 5. QRS complex: _____ +1. ST elevation: _____

+2. ST depression: _____ +3. Pathologic Q waves: _____ Interpretation: _____

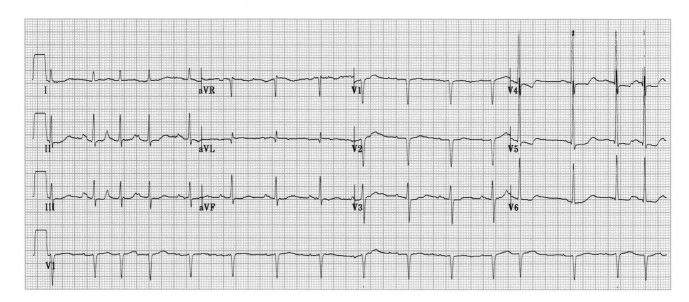

74

1. Rate: _____ 2. Rhythm: _____ 3. P wave: _____

4. PR Interval: _____ 5. QRS complex: _____ +1. ST elevation: _____

+2. ST depression: _____ +3. Pathologic Q waves: _____ Interpretation: _____

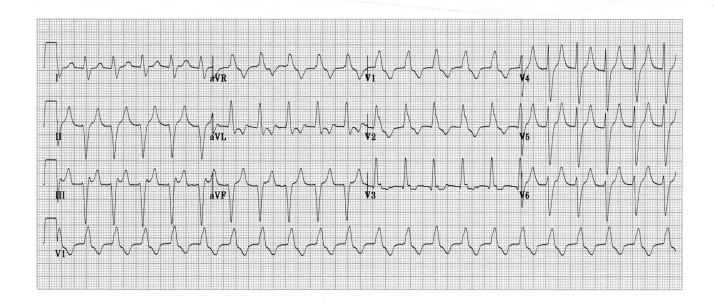

75

1. Rate: _____

2. Rhythm: _____

3. P wave: _____

4. PR Interval: _____

5. QRS complex: _____

+1. ST elevation: _____

+2. ST depression: _____

+3. Pathologic Q waves: _____

Interpretation: _____

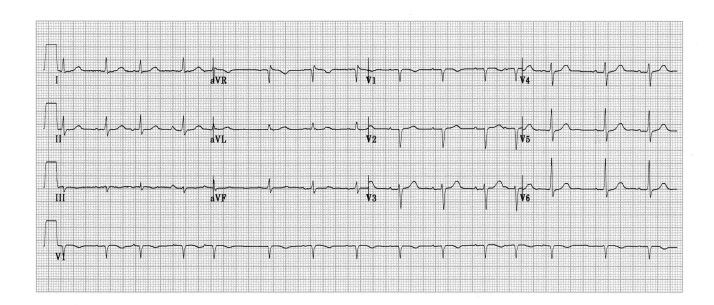

76

1. Rate: _____

2. Rhythm: _____

3. P wave: _____

4. PR Interval: _____

5. QRS complex: _____

+1. ST elevation: _____

+2. ST depression: _____

+3. Pathologic Q waves: _____

Interpretation: _____

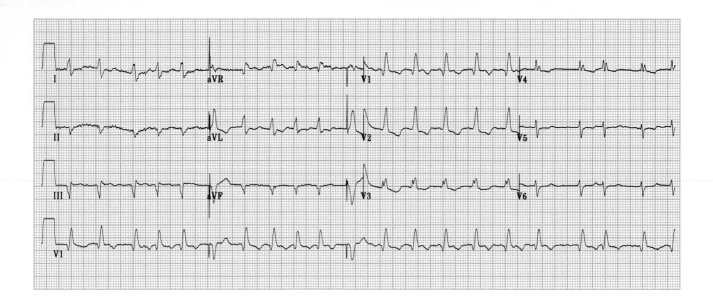

77

1. Rate: _____

2. Rhythm: _____

3. P wave: _____

4. PR Interval: _____

5. QRS complex: _____

+1. ST elevation: _____

+2. ST depression: _____

+3. Pathologic Q waves: _____

Interpretation: _____

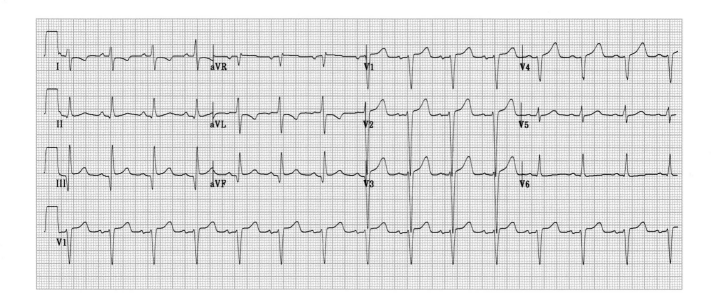

78

1. Rate: _____

2. Rhythm: _____

3. P wave: _____

4. PR Interval: _____

5. QRS complex: _____

+1. ST elevation: _____

+2. ST depression: _____

+3. Pathologic Q waves: _____

Interpretation: _____

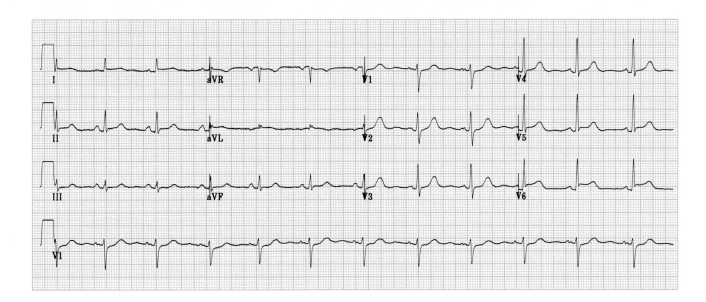

79

1. Rate: _____

2. Rhythm: _____

3. P wave: _____

4. PR Interval: _____

5. QRS complex: _____

+1. ST elevation: _____

+2. ST depression: _____

+3. Pathologic Q waves: _____

Interpretation: _____

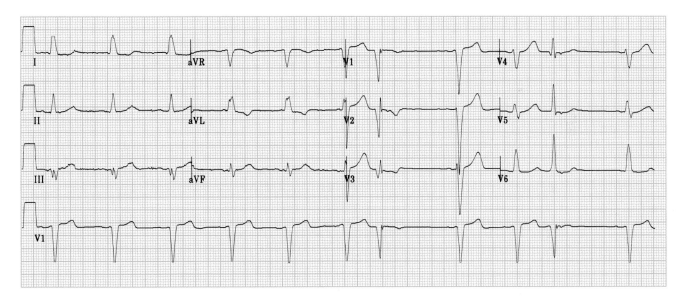

80

1. Rate: _____

2. Rhythm: _____

3. P wave: _____

4. PR Interval: _____

5. QRS complex: _____

+1. ST elevation: _____

+2. ST depression: _____

+3. Pathologic Q waves: _____

Interpretation: _____

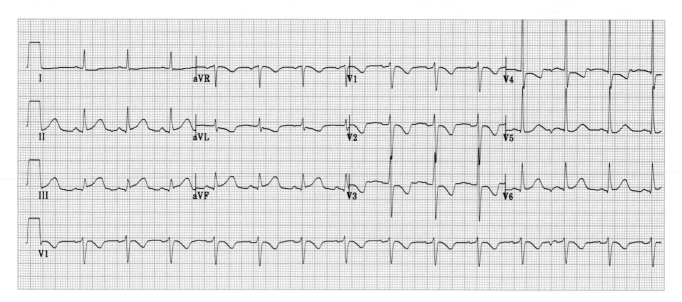

81

1. Rate: _____

2. Rhythm: _____

3. P wave: _____

4. PR Interval: _____

5. QRS complex: _____

+1. ST elevation: _____

+2. ST depression: _____

+3. Pathologic Q waves: _____

Interpretation: _____

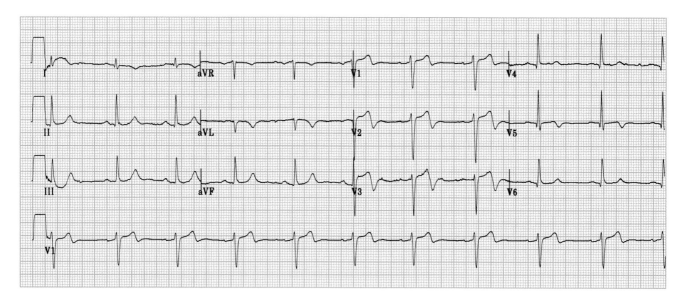

82

1. Rate: _____

2. Rhythm: _____

3. P wave: _____

4. PR Interval: _____

5. QRS complex: _____

+1. ST elevation: _____

+2. ST depression: _____

+3. Pathologic Q waves: _____

Interpretation: _____

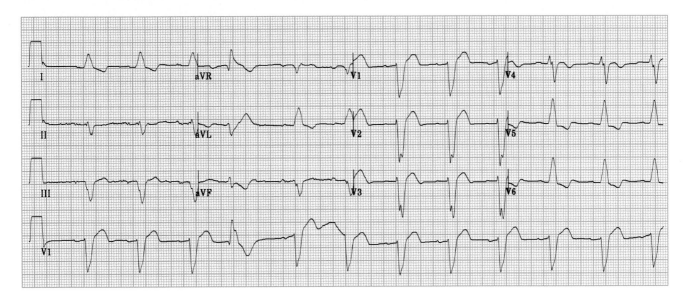

83

1. Rate: _____

2. Rhythm: _____

3. P wave: _____

4. PR Interval: _____

5. QRS complex: _____

+1. ST elevation: _____

+2. ST depression: _____

+3. Pathologic Q waves: _____

Interpretation: _____

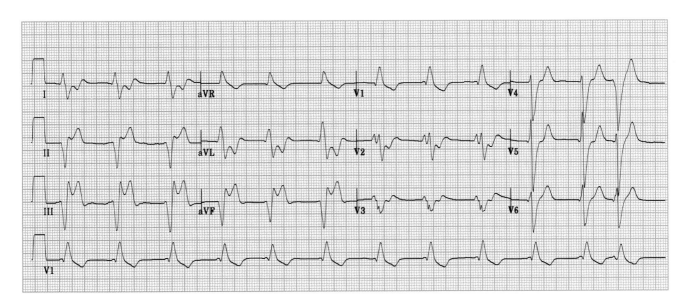

84

1. Rate: _____

2. Rhythm: _____

3. P wave: _____

4. PR Interval: _____

5. QRS complex: _____

+1. ST elevation: _____

+2. ST depression: _____

+3. Pathologic Q waves: _____

Interpretation: _____

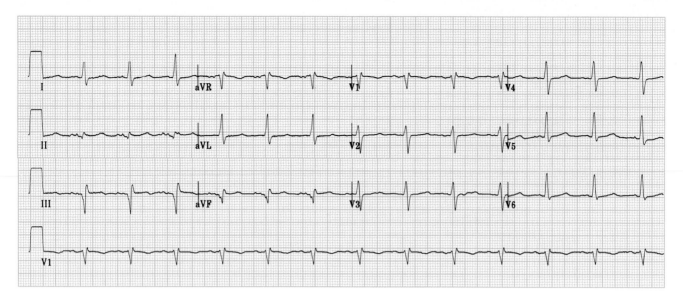

85

1. Rate: _____

2. Rhythm: _____

3. P wave: _____

4. PR Interval: _____

5. QRS complex: _____

+1. ST elevation: _____

+2. ST depression: _____

+3. Pathologic Q waves: _____

Interpretation: _____

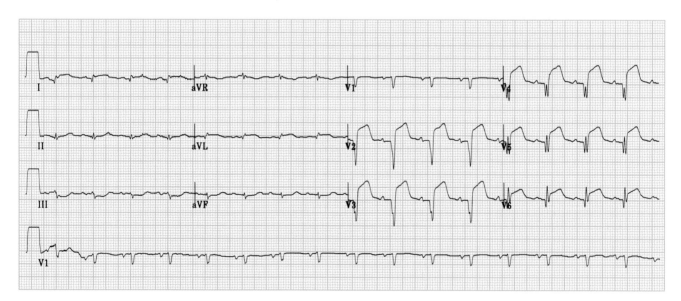

86

1. Rate: _____

2. Rhythm: _____

3. P wave: _____

4. PR Interval: _____

5. QRS complex: _____

+1. ST elevation: _____

+2. ST depression: _____

+3. Pathologic Q waves: _____

Interpretation: _____

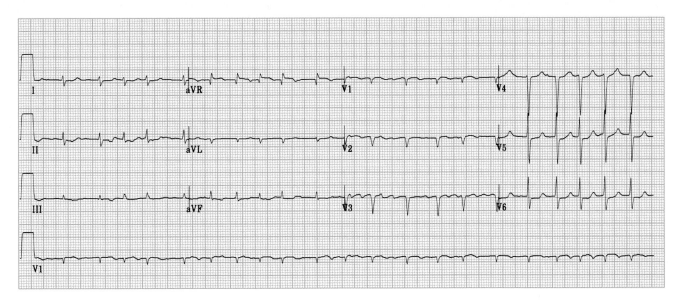

87

1. Rate: _____

2. Rhythm: _____

3. P wave: _____

4. PR Interval: _____

5. QRS complex: _____

+1. ST elevation: _____

+2. ST depression: _____

+3. Pathologic Q waves: _____

Interpretation: _____

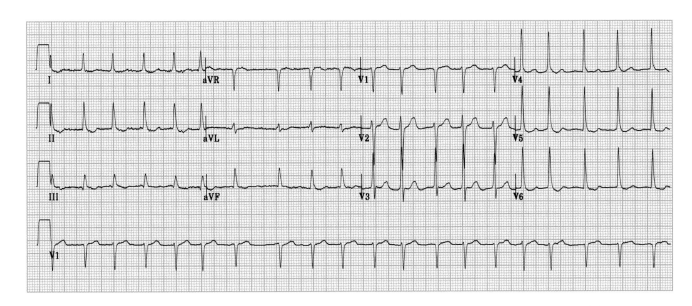

88

1. Rate: _____

2. Rhythm: _____

3. P wave: _____

4. PR Interval: _____

5. QRS complex: _____

+1. ST elevation: _____

+2. ST depression: _____

+3. Pathologic Q waves: _____

Interpretation: _____

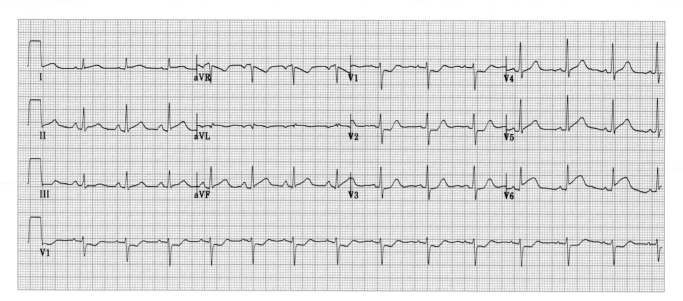

89

1. Rate: _____

2. Rhythm: _____

3. P wave: _____

4. PR Interval: _____

5. QRS complex: _____

+1. ST elevation: _____

+2. ST depression: _____

+3. Pathologic Q waves: _____

Interpretation: _____

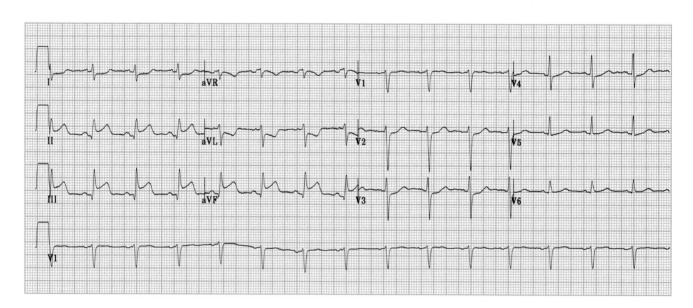

90

1. Rate: _____

2. Rhythm: _____

3. P wave: _____

4. PR Interval: _____

5. QRS complex: _____

+1. ST elevation: _____

+2. ST depression: _____

+3. Pathologic Q waves: _____

Interpretation: _____

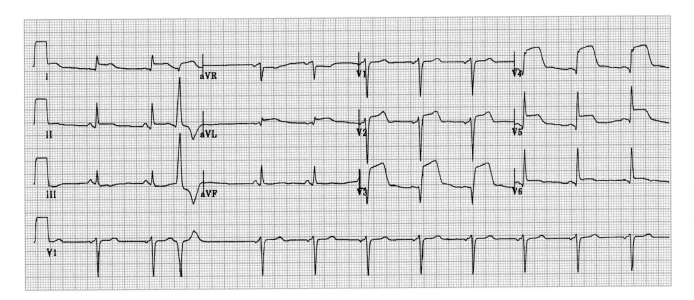

91

1. Rate: _____

2. Rhythm: _____

3. P wave: _____

4. PR Interval: _____

5. QRS complex: _____

+1. ST elevation: _____

+2. ST depression: _____

+3. Pathologic Q waves: _____

Interpretation: _____

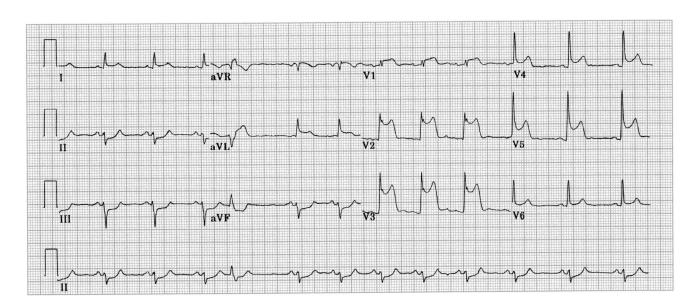

92

1. Rate: _____

2. Rhythm: _____

3. P wave: _____

4. PR Interval: _____

5. QRS complex: _____

+1. ST elevation: _____

+2. ST depression: _____

+3. Pathologic Q waves: _____

Interpretation: _____

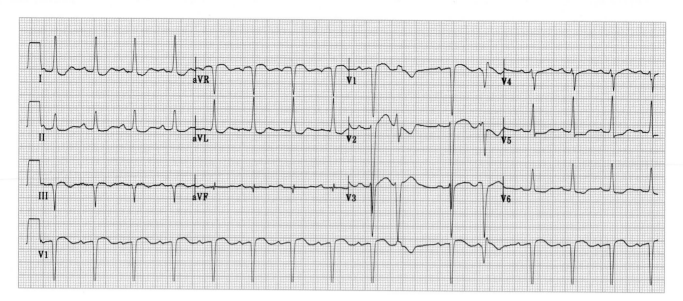

93

1. Rate: _____   2. Rhythm: _____   3. P wave: _____

4. PR Interval: _____   5. QRS complex: _____   +1. ST elevation: _____

+2. ST depression: _____   +3. Pathologic Q waves: _____   Interpretation: _____

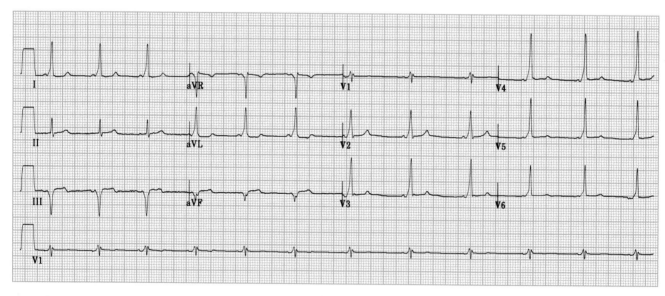

94

1. Rate: _____   2. Rhythm: _____   3. P wave: _____

4. PR Interval: _____   5. QRS complex: _____   +1. ST elevation: _____

+2. ST depression: _____   +3. Pathologic Q waves: _____   Interpretation: _____

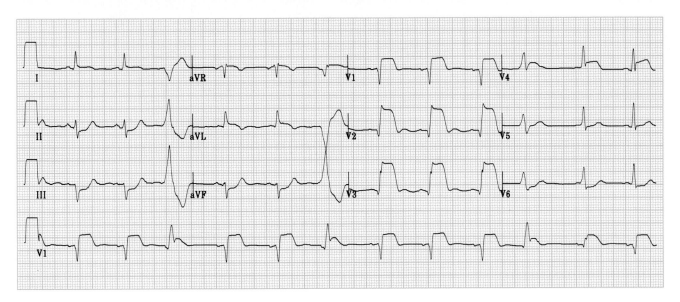

95

1. Rate: _____

2. Rhythm: _____

3. P wave: _____

4. PR Interval: _____

5. QRS complex: _____

+1. ST elevation: _____

+2. ST depression: _____

+3. Pathologic Q waves: _____

Interpretation: _____

96

1. Rate: _____

2. Rhythm: _____

3. P wave: _____

4. PR Interval: _____

5. QRS complex: _____

+1. ST elevation: _____

+2. ST depression: _____

+3. Pathologic Q waves: _____

Interpretation: _____

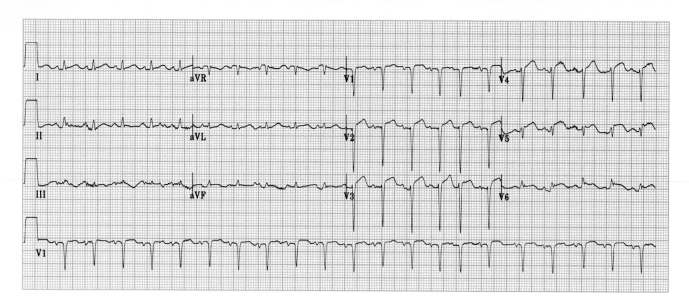

97

1. Rate: _____ 2. Rhythm:_____ 3. P wave: _____

4. PR Interval: _____ 5. QRS complex: _____ +1. ST elevation: _____

+2. ST depression: _____ +3. Pathologic Q waves: _____ Interpretation: _____

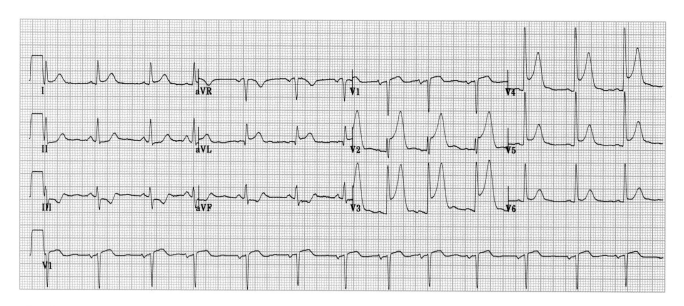

98

1. Rate: _____ 2. Rhythm:_____ 3. P wave: _____

4. PR Interval: _____ 5. QRS complex: _____ +1. ST elevation: _____

+2. ST depression: _____ +3. Pathologic Q waves: _____ Interpretation: _____

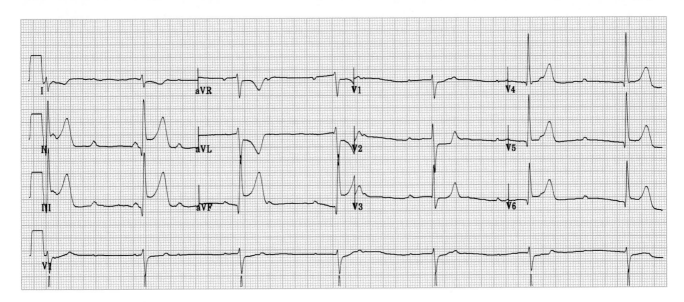

99

1. Rate: _____
4. PR Interval: _____
+2. ST depression: _____

2. Rhythm: _____
5. QRS complex: _____
+3. Pathologic Q waves: _____

3. P wave: _____
+1. ST elevation: _____
Interpretation: _____

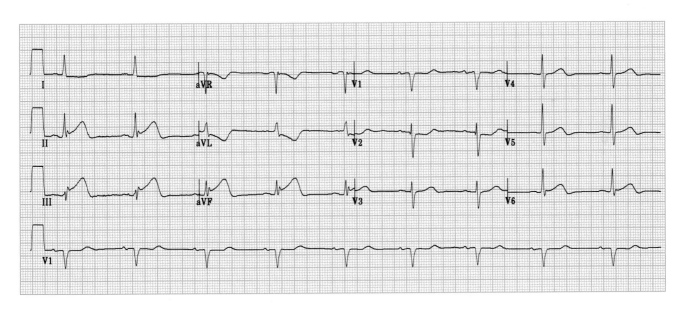

100

1. Rate: _____
4. PR Interval: _____
+2. ST depression: _____

2. Rhythm: _____
5. QRS complex: _____
+3. Pathologic Q waves: _____

3. P wave: _____
+1. ST elevation: _____
Interpretation: _____

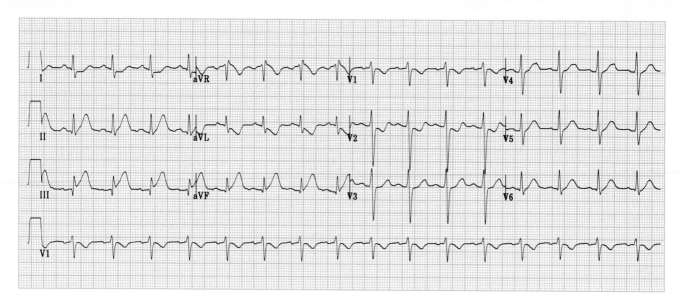

101

1. Rate: _____   2. Rhythm: _____   3. P wave: _____

4. PR Interval: _____   5. QRS complex: _____   +1. ST elevation: _____

+2. ST depression: _____   +3. Pathologic Q waves: _____   Interpretation: _____

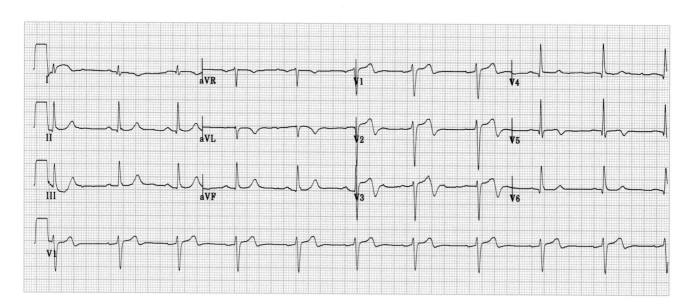

102

1. Rate: _____   2. Rhythm: _____   3. P wave: _____

4. PR Interval: _____   5. QRS complex: _____   +1. ST elevation: _____

+2. ST depression: _____   +3. Pathologic Q waves: _____   Interpretation: _____

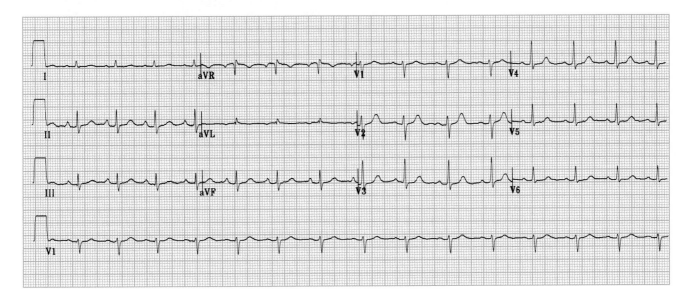

103

1. Rate: _____

2. Rhythm: _____

3. P wave: _____

4. PR Interval: _____

5. QRS complex: _____

+1. ST elevation: _____

+2. ST depression: _____

+3. Pathologic Q waves: _____

Interpretation: _____

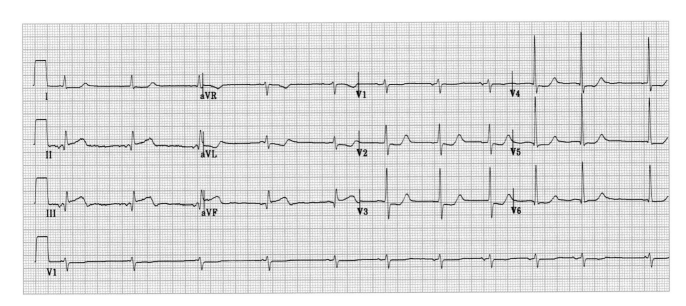

104

1. Rate: _____

2. Rhythm: _____

3. P wave: _____

4. PR Interval: _____

5. QRS complex: _____

+1. ST elevation: _____

+2. ST depression: _____

+3. Pathologic Q waves: _____

Interpretation: _____

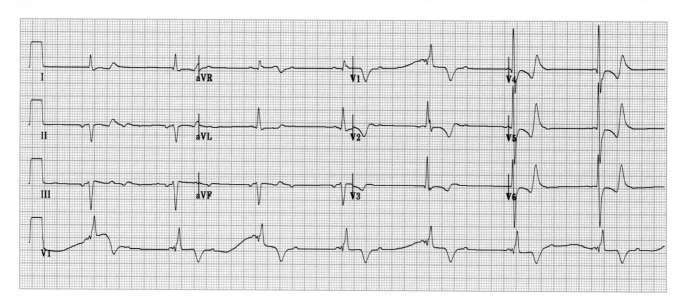

105

1. Rate: _____   2. Rhythm: _____   3. P wave: _____

4. PR Interval: _____   5. QRS complex: _____   +1. ST elevation: _____

+2. ST depression: _____   +3. Pathologic Q waves: _____   Interpretation: _____

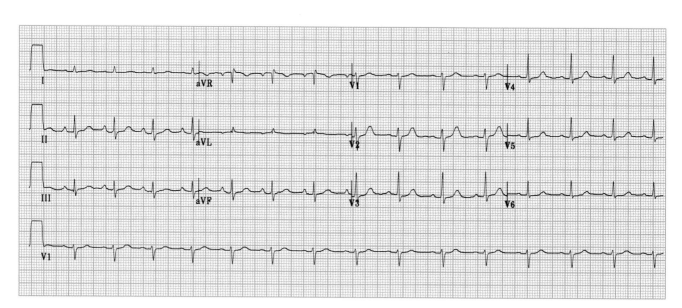

106

1. Rate: _____   2. Rhythm: _____   3. P wave: _____

4. PR Interval: _____   5. QRS complex: _____   +1. ST elevation: _____

+2. ST depression: _____   +3. Pathologic Q waves: _____   Interpretation: _____

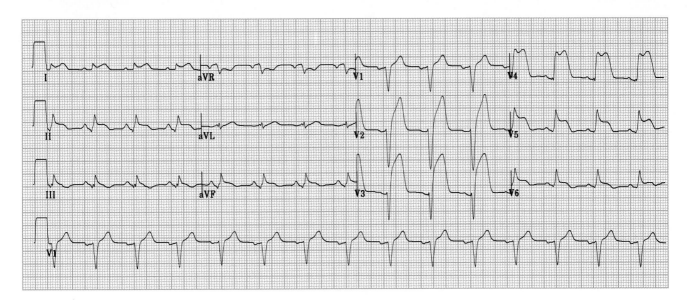

107

1. Rate: _____

2. Rhythm: _____

3. P wave: _____

4. PR Interval: _____

5. QRS complex: _____

+1. ST elevation: _____

+2. ST depression: _____

+3. Pathologic Q waves: _____

Interpretation: _____

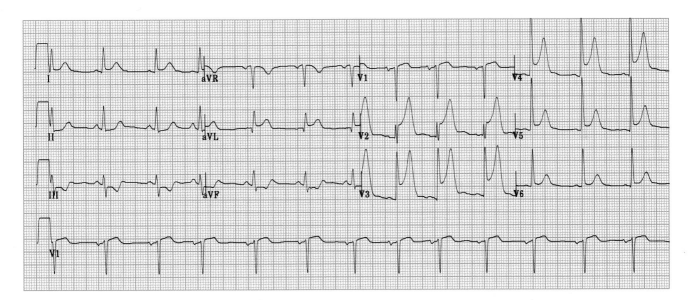

108

1. Rate: _____

2. Rhythm: _____

3. P wave: _____

4. PR Interval: _____

5. QRS complex: _____

+1. ST elevation: _____

+2. ST depression: _____

+3. Pathologic Q waves: _____

Interpretation: _____

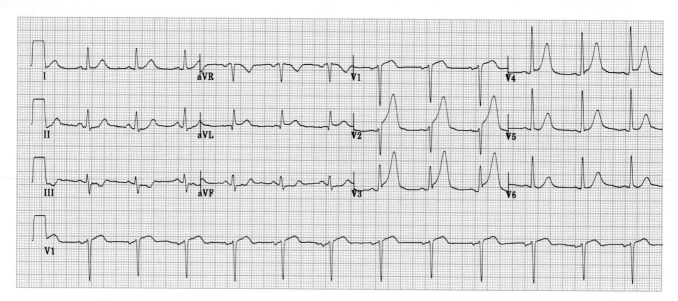

109

1. Rate: _____ 2. Rhythm: _____ 3. P wave: _____

4. PR Interval: _____ 5. QRS complex: _____ +1. ST elevation: _____

+2. ST depression: _____ +3. Pathologic Q waves: _____ Interpretation: _____

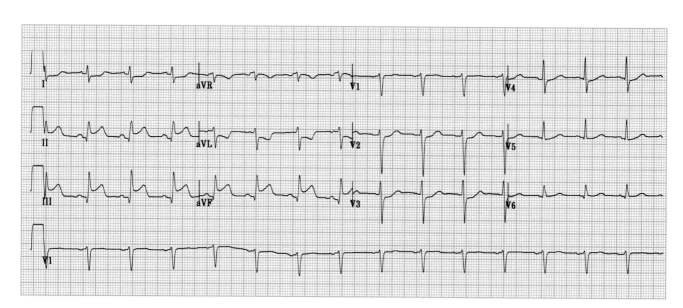

110

1. Rate: _____ 2. Rhythm: _____ 3. P wave: _____

4. PR Interval: _____ 5. QRS complex: _____ +1. ST elevation: _____

+2. ST depression: _____ +3. Pathologic Q waves: _____ Interpretation: _____

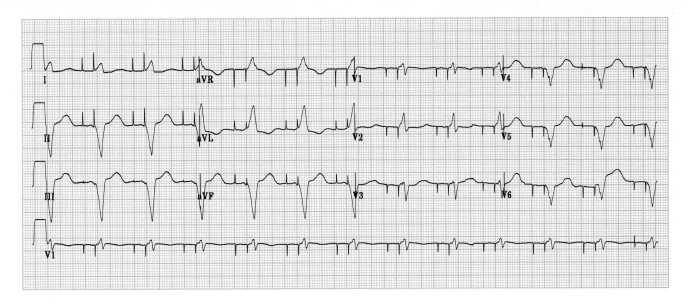

111

1. Rate: _____

2. Rhythm: _____

3. P wave: _____

4. PR Interval: _____

5. QRS complex: _____

+1. ST elevation: _____

+2. ST depression: _____

+3. Pathologic Q waves: _____

Interpretation: _____

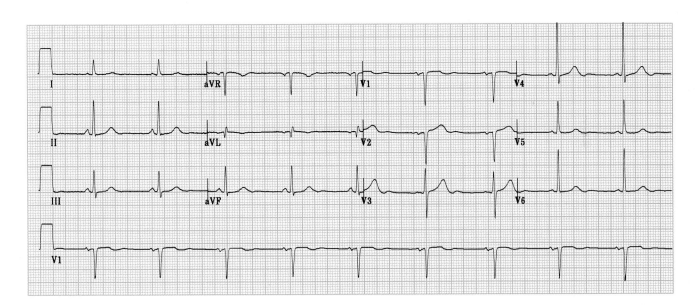

112

1. Rate: _____

2. Rhythm: _____

3. P wave: _____

4. PR Interval: _____

5. QRS complex: _____

+1. ST elevation: _____

+2. ST depression: _____

+3. Pathologic Q waves: _____

Interpretation: _____

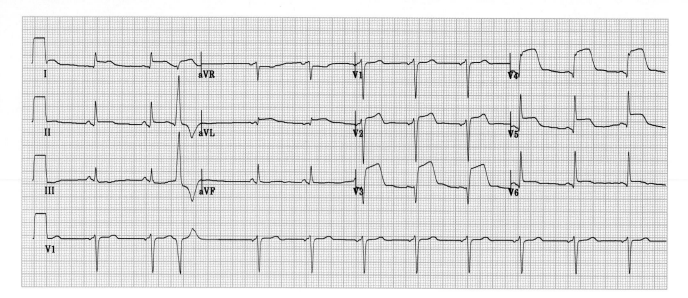

113

1. Rate: _____

2. Rhythm: _____

3. P wave: _____

4. PR Interval: _____

5. QRS complex: _____

+1. ST elevation: _____

+2. ST depression: _____

+3. Pathologic Q waves: _____

Interpretation: _____

114

1. Rate: _____

2. Rhythm: _____

3. P wave: _____

4. PR Interval: _____

5. QRS complex: _____

+1. ST elevation: _____

+2. ST depression: _____

+3. Pathologic Q waves: _____

Interpretation: _____

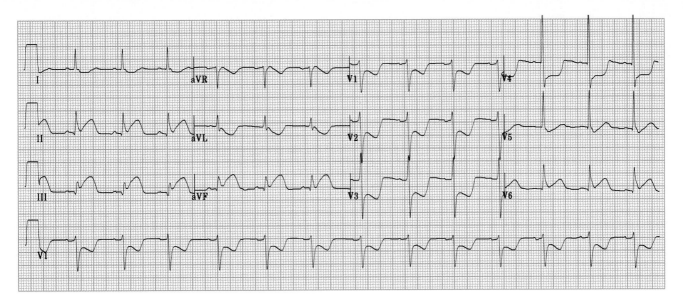

115

1. Rate: _____

2. Rhythm: _____

3. P wave: _____

4. PR Interval: _____

5. QRS complex: _____

+1. ST elevation: _____

+2. ST depression: _____

+3. Pathologic Q waves: _____

Interpretation: _____

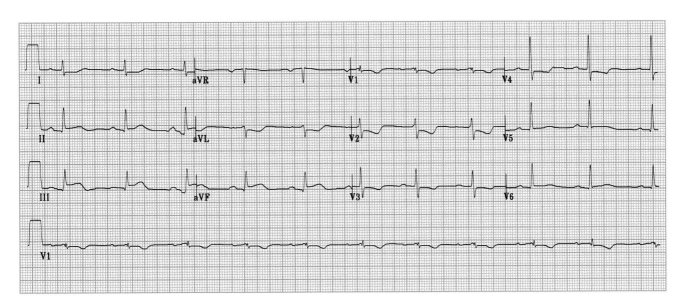

116

1. Rate: _____

2. Rhythm: _____

3. P wave: _____

4. PR Interval: _____

5. QRS complex: _____

+1. ST elevation: _____

+2. ST depression: _____

+3. Pathologic Q waves: _____

Interpretation: _____

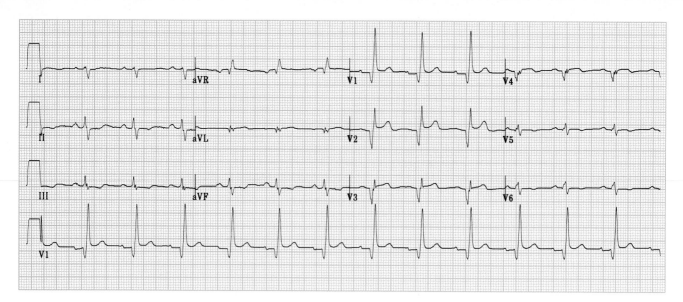

117

1. Rate: _____   2. Rhythm: _____   3. P wave: _____

4. PR Interval: _____   5. QRS complex: _____   +1. ST elevation: _____

+2. ST depression: _____   +3. Pathologic Q waves: _____   Interpretation: _____

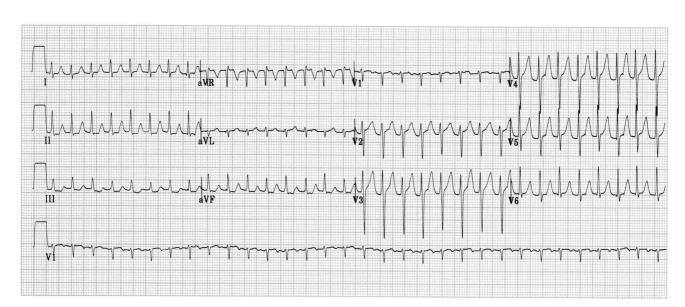

118

1. Rate: _____   2. Rhythm: _____   3. P wave: _____

4. PR Interval: _____   5. QRS complex: _____   +1. ST elevation: _____

+2. ST depression: _____   +3. Pathologic Q waves: _____   Interpretation: _____

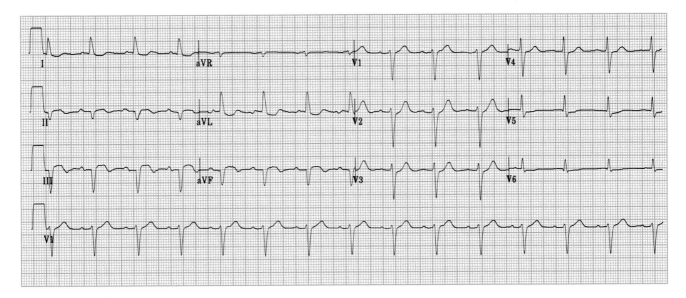

119

1. Rate: _____

4. PR Interval: _____

+2. ST depression: _____

2. Rhythm: _____

5. QRS complex: _____

+3. Pathologic Q waves: _____

3. P wave: _____

+1. ST elevation: _____

Interpretation: _____

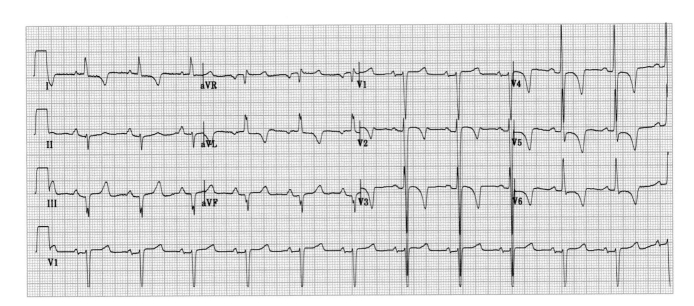

120

1. Rate: _____

4. PR Interval: _____

+2. ST depression: _____

2. Rhythm: _____

5. QRS complex: _____

+3. Pathologic Q waves: _____

3. P wave: _____

+1. ST elevation: _____

Interpretation: _____

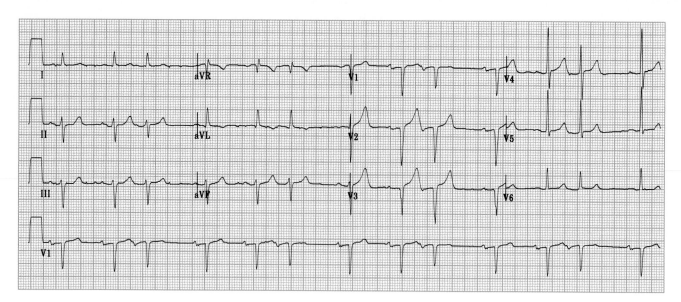

121

1. Rate: _____

2. Rhythm: _____

3. P wave: _____

4. PR Interval: _____

5. QRS complex: _____

+1. ST elevation: _____

+2. ST depression: _____

+3. Pathologic Q waves: _____

Interpretation: _____

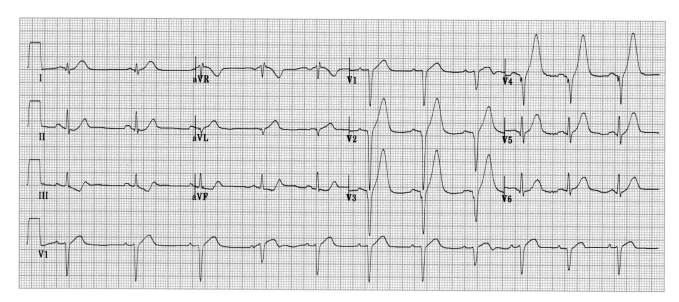

122

1. Rate: _____

2. Rhythm: _____

3. P wave: _____

4. PR Interval: _____

5. QRS complex: _____

+1. ST elevation: _____

+2. ST depression: _____

+3. Pathologic Q waves: _____

Interpretation: _____

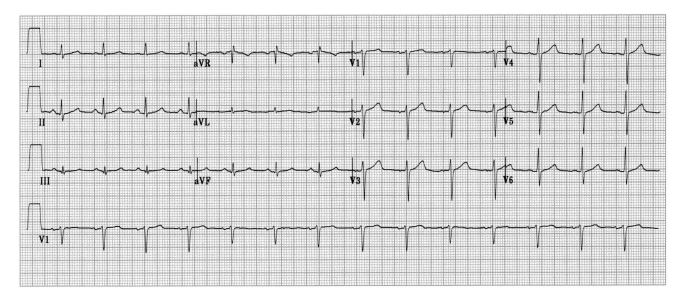

123

1. Rate: _____

2. Rhythm: _____

3. P wave: _____

4. PR Interval: _____

5. QRS complex: _____

+1. ST elevation: _____

+2. ST depression: _____

+3. Pathologic Q waves: _____

Interpretation: _____

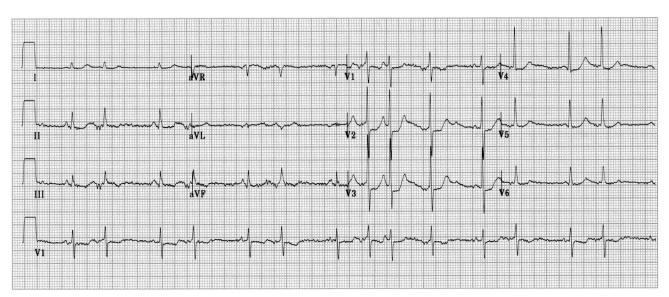

124

1. Rate: _____

2. Rhythm: _____

3. P wave: _____

4. PR Interval: _____

5. QRS complex: _____

+1. ST elevation: _____

+2. ST depression: _____

+3. Pathologic Q waves: _____

Interpretation: _____

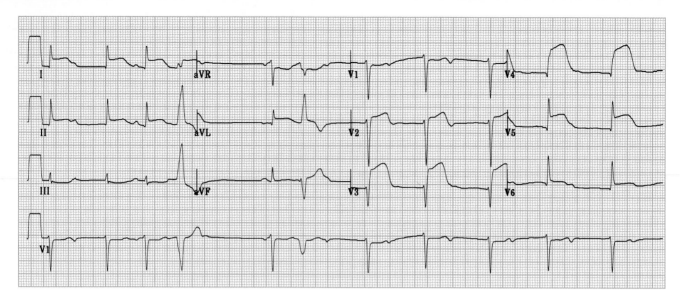

125

1. Rate: _____   2. Rhythm: _____   3. P wave: _____

4. PR Interval: _____   5. QRS complex: _____   +1. ST elevation: _____

+2. ST depression: _____   +3. Pathologic Q waves: _____   Interpretation: _____

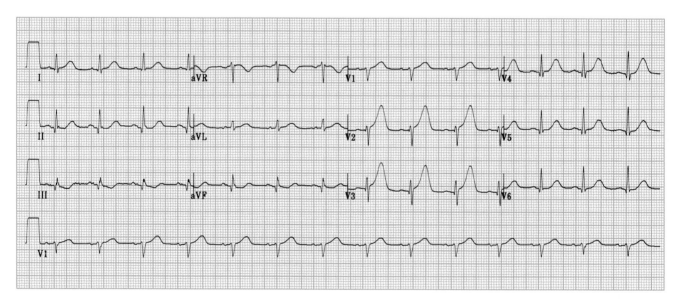

126

1. Rate: _____   2. Rhythm: _____   3. P wave: _____

4. PR Interval: _____   5. QRS complex: _____   +1. ST elevation: _____

+2. ST depression: _____   +3. Pathologic Q waves: _____   Interpretation: _____

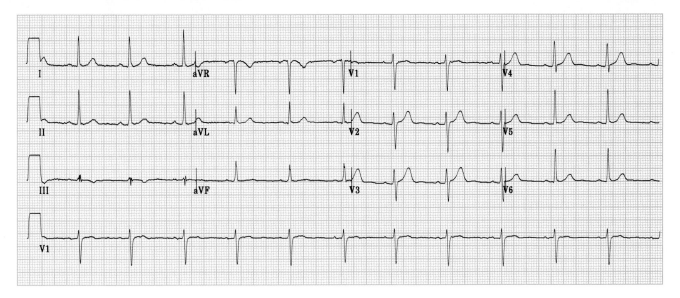

127

1. Rate: _____

2. Rhythm: _____

3. P wave: _____

4. PR Interval: _____

5. QRS complex: _____

+1. ST elevation: _____

+2. ST depression: _____

+3. Pathologic Q waves: _____

Interpretation: _____

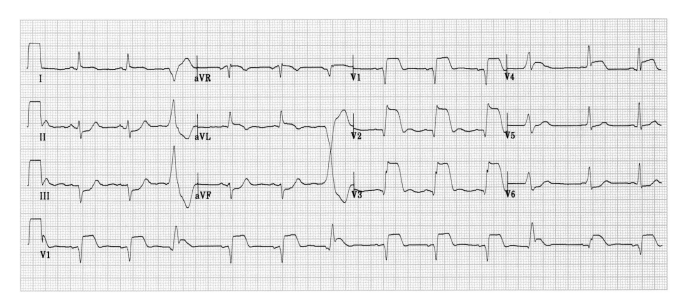

128

1. Rate: _____

2. Rhythm: _____

3. P wave: _____

4. PR Interval: _____

5. QRS complex: _____

+1. ST elevation: _____

+2. ST depression: _____

+3. Pathologic Q waves: _____

Interpretation: _____

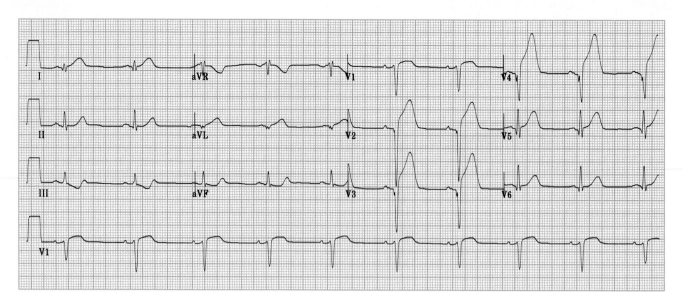

129

1. Rate: _____

2. Rhythm: _____

3. P wave: _____

4. PR Interval: _____

5. QRS complex: _____

+1. ST elevation: _____

+2. ST depression: _____

+3. Pathologic Q waves: _____

Interpretation: _____

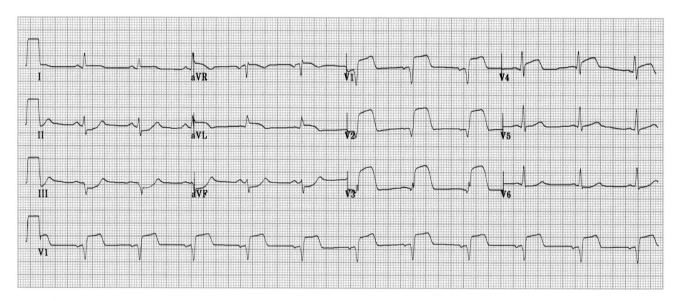

130

1. Rate: _____

2. Rhythm: _____

3. P wave: _____

4. PR Interval: _____

5. QRS complex: _____

+1. ST elevation: _____

+2. ST depression: _____

+3. Pathologic Q waves: _____

Interpretation: _____

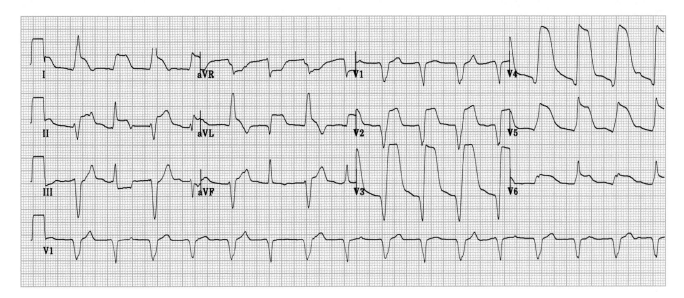

131

1. Rate: _____

2. Rhythm: _____

3. P wave: _____

4. PR Interval: _____

5. QRS complex: _____

+1. ST elevation: _____

+2. ST depression: _____

+3. Pathologic Q waves: _____

Interpretation: _____

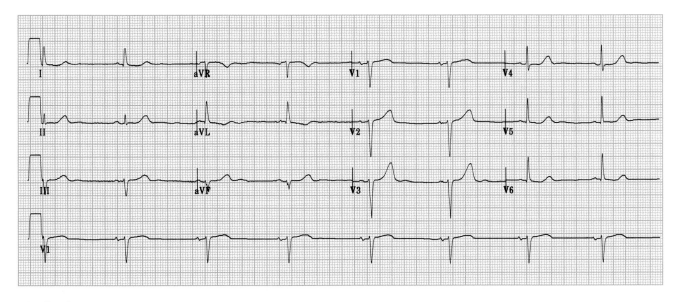

132

1. Rate: _____

2. Rhythm: _____

3. P wave: _____

4. PR Interval: _____

5. QRS complex: _____

+1. ST elevation: _____

+2. ST depression: _____

+3. Pathologic Q waves: _____

Interpretation: _____

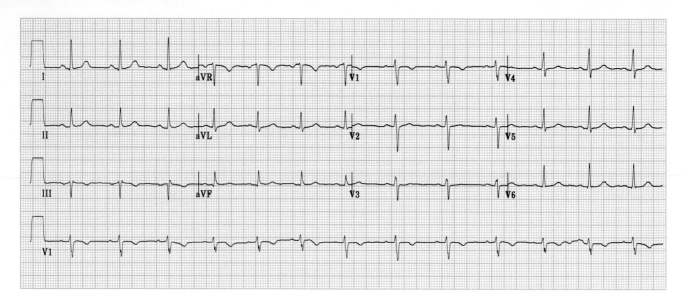

133

1. Rate: _____

2. Rhythm: _____

3. P wave: _____

4. PR Interval: _____

5. QRS complex: _____

+1. ST elevation: _____

+2. ST depression: _____

+3. Pathologic Q waves: _____

Interpretation: _____

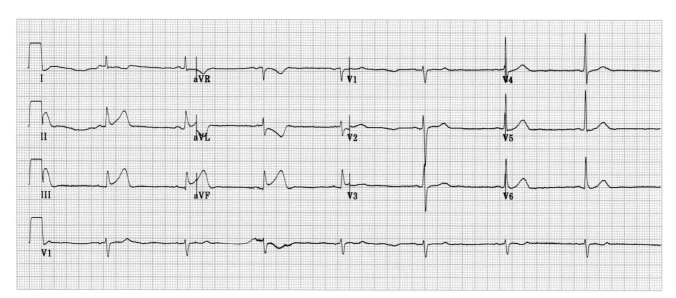

134

1. Rate: _____

2. Rhythm: _____

3. P wave: _____

4. PR Interval: _____

5. QRS complex: _____

+1. ST elevation: _____

+2. ST depression: _____

+3. Pathologic Q waves: _____

Interpretation: _____

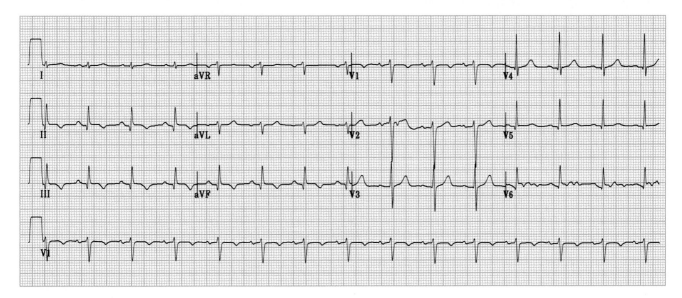

135

1. Rate: _____

4. PR Interval: _____

+2. ST depression: _____

2. Rhythm: _____

5. QRS complex: _____

+3. Pathologic Q waves: _____

3. P wave: _____

+1. ST elevation: _____

Interpretation: _____

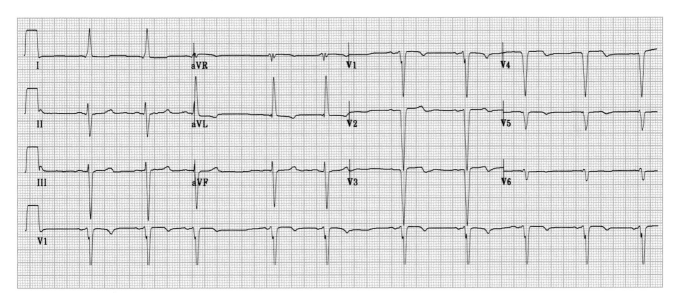

136

1. Rate: _____

4. PR Interval: _____

+2. ST depression: _____

2. Rhythm: _____

5. QRS complex: _____

+3. Pathologic Q waves: _____

3. P wave: _____

+1. ST elevation: _____

Interpretation: _____

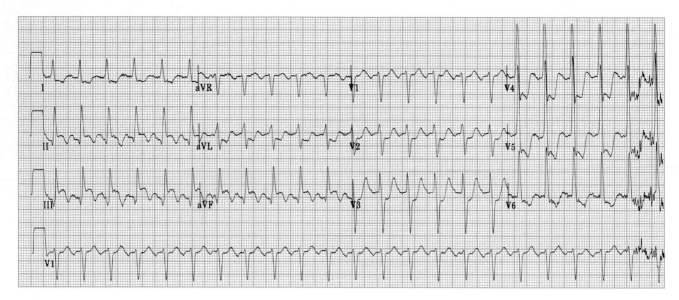

137

1. Rate: _____

2. Rhythm: _____

3. P wave: _____

4. PR Interval: _____

5. QRS complex: _____

+1. ST elevation: _____

+2. ST depression: _____

+3. Pathologic Q waves: _____

Interpretation: _____

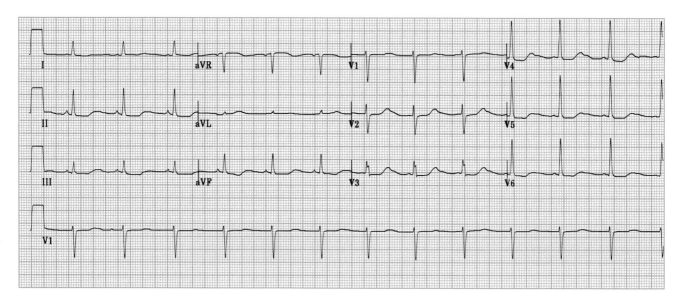

138

1. Rate: _____

2. Rhythm: _____

3. P wave: _____

4. PR Interval: _____

5. QRS complex: _____

+1. ST elevation: _____

+2. ST depression: _____

+3. Pathologic Q waves: _____

Interpretation: _____

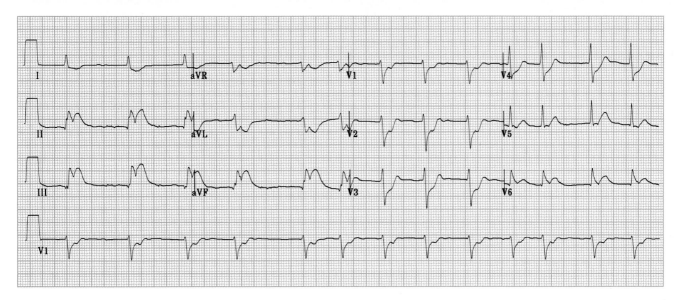

139

1. Rate: _____

2. Rhythm: _____

3. P wave: _____

4. PR Interval: _____

5. QRS complex: _____

+1. ST elevation: _____

+2. ST depression: _____

+3. Pathologic Q waves: _____

Interpretation: _____

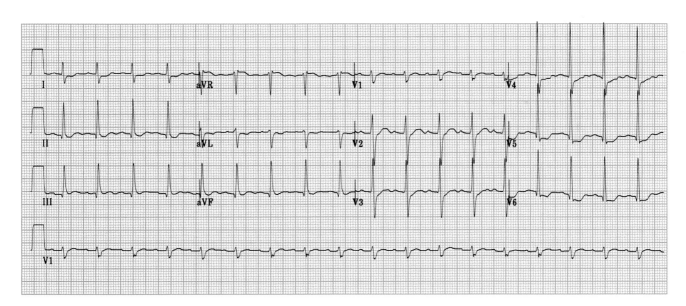

140

1. Rate: _____

2. Rhythm: _____

3. P wave: _____

4. PR Interval: _____

5. QRS complex: _____

+1. ST elevation: _____

+2. ST depression: _____

+3. Pathologic Q waves: _____

Interpretation: _____

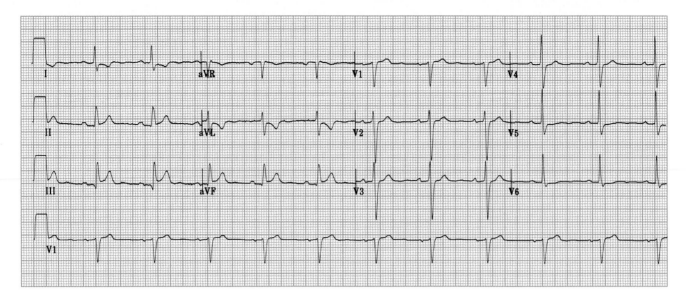

141

1. Rate: _____

2. Rhythm: _____

3. P wave: _____

4. PR Interval: _____

5. QRS complex: _____

+1. ST elevation: _____

+2. ST depression: _____

+3. Pathologic Q waves: _____

Interpretation: _____

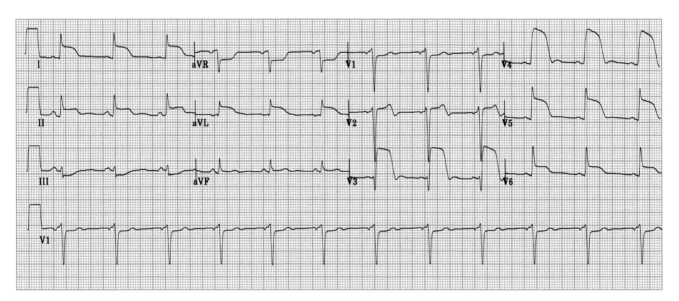

142

1. Rate: _____

2. Rhythm: _____

3. P wave: _____

4. PR Interval: _____

5. QRS complex: _____

+1. ST elevation: _____

+2. ST depression: _____

+3. Pathologic Q waves: _____

Interpretation: _____

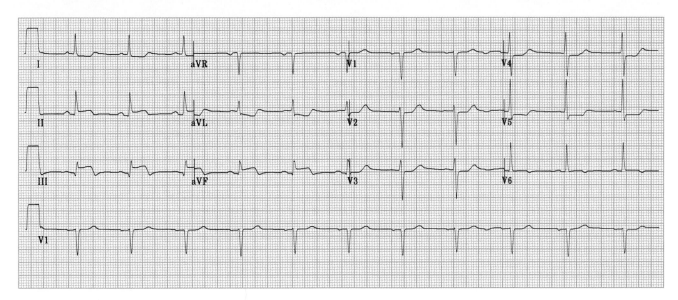

143

1. Rate: _____ 2. Rhythm: _____ 3. P wave: _____

4. PR Interval: _____ 5. QRS complex: _____ +1. ST elevation: _____

+2. ST depression: _____ +3. Pathologic Q waves: _____ Interpretation: _____

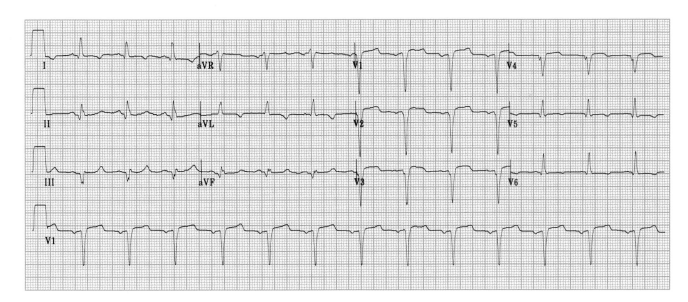

144

1. Rate: _____ 2. Rhythm: _____ 3. P wave: _____

4. PR Interval: _____ 5. QRS complex: _____ +1. ST elevation: _____

+2. ST depression: _____ +3. Pathologic Q waves: _____ Interpretation: _____

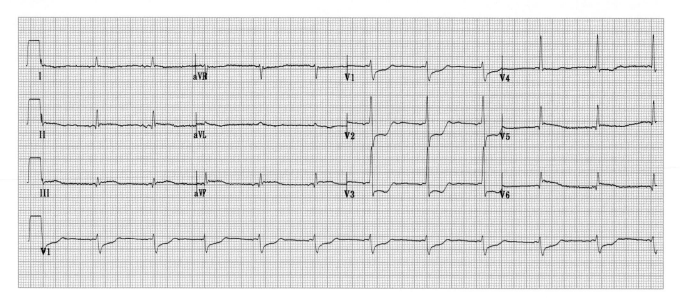

145

1. Rate: _____   2. Rhythm: _____   3. P wave: _____

4. PR Interval: _____   5. QRS complex: _____   +1. ST elevation: _____

+2. ST depression: _____   +3. Pathologic Q waves: _____   Interpretation: _____

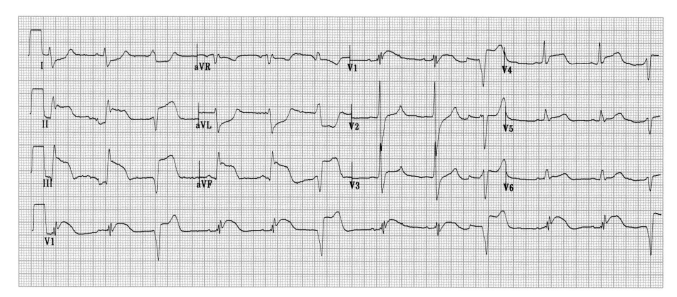

146

1. Rate: _____   2. Rhythm: _____   3. P wave: _____

4. PR Interval: _____   5. QRS complex: _____   +1. ST elevation: _____

+2. ST depression: _____   +3. Pathologic Q waves: _____   Interpretation: _____

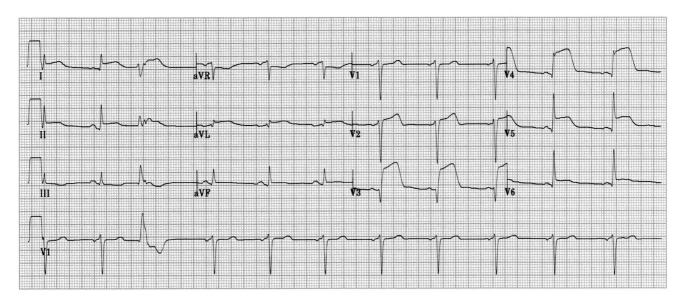

147

1. Rate: _____

2. Rhythm: _____

3. P wave: _____

4. PR Interval: _____

5. QRS complex: _____

+1. ST elevation: _____

+2. ST depression: _____

+3. Pathologic Q waves: _____

Interpretation: _____

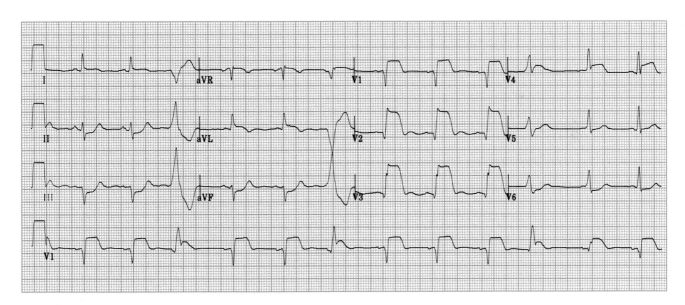

148

1. Rate: _____

2. Rhythm: _____

3. P wave: _____

4. PR Interval: _____

5. QRS complex: _____

+1. ST elevation: _____

+2. ST depression: _____

+3. Pathologic Q waves: _____

Interpretation: _____

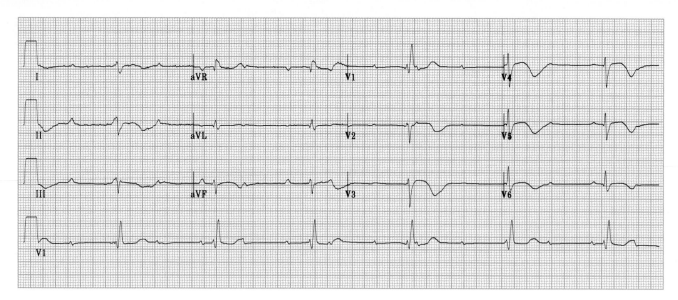

149

1. Rate: _____   2. Rhythm: _____   3. P wave: _____

4. PR Interval: _____   5. QRS complex: _____   +1. ST elevation: _____

+2. ST depression: _____   +3. Pathologic Q waves: _____   Interpretation: _____

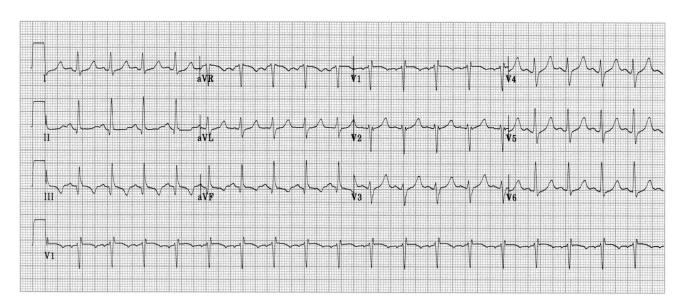

150

1. Rate: _____   2. Rhythm: _____   3. P wave: _____

4. PR Interval: _____   5. QRS complex: _____   +1. ST elevation: _____

+2. ST depression: _____   +3. Pathologic Q waves: _____   Interpretation: _____

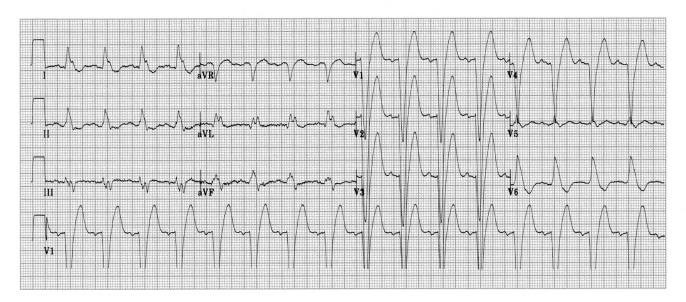

151

1. Rate: _____

2. Rhythm: _____

3. P wave: _____

4. PR Interval: _____

5. QRS complex: _____

+1. ST elevation: _____

+2. ST depression: _____

+3. Pathologic Q waves: _____

Interpretation: _____

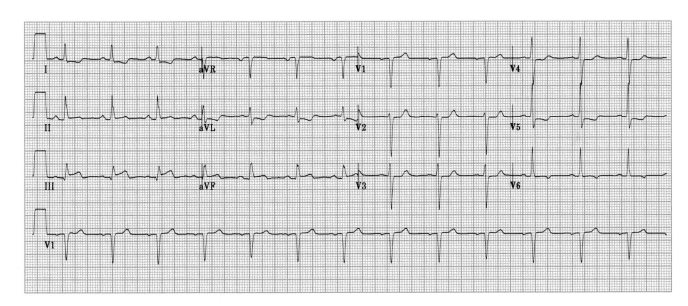

152

1. Rate: _____

2. Rhythm: _____

3. P wave: _____

4. PR Interval: _____

5. QRS complex: _____

+1. ST elevation: _____

+2. ST depression: _____

+3. Pathologic Q waves: _____

Interpretation: _____

Appendix 1

Answers to Review Questions

Chapters 1–17

Chapter 1

1. c
2. b
3. a
4. c
5. a
6. b
7. d
8. c
9. c
10. c

Chapter 2

1. b
2. b
3. b
4. d
5. a
6. c
7. b
8. d
9. a
10. b

Chapter 3

1. c
2. a
3. c
4. d
5. a
6. b
7. b
8. a
9. b
10. a

Chapter 4

1. a
2. d
3. d
4. c
5. c
6. b
7. b
8. c
9. a
10. d

CHAPTER 5

1. b
2. c
3. d
4. b
5. d
6. b
7. a
8. c
9. d
10. a

CHAPTER 6

1. a
2. d
3. c
4. b
5. d
6. b
7. a
8. d
9. b
10. c
11. a
12. d

CHAPTER 7

1. c
2. a
3. b
4. d
5. c
6. d
7. b
8. c
9. a
10. d

11. a
12. b

CHAPTER 8

1. a
2. d
3. c
4. c
5. b
6. a
7. a
8. a
9. d
10. b
11. b
12. a

CHAPTER 9

1. c
2. d
3. a
4. b
5. c
6. b
7. a
8. c
9. d
10. c
11. c
12. a

CHAPTER 10

1. b
2. a
3. c
4. d
5. a

6. a
7. c
8. c
9. b
10. d
11. b
12. a

Chapter 11

1. b
2. a
3. c
4. d
5. c
6. a
7. b
8. d
9. a
10. b
11. b
12. a

Chapter 12

1. d
2. a
3. d
4. a
5. a
6. a
7. c
8. a
9. d
10. b
11. a
12. b

Chapter 13

1. c
2. a
3. d
4. d
5. c
6. c
7. b
8. c
9. b
10. c
11. b
12. b

Chapter 14

1. b
2. d
3. c
4. a
5. c
6. b
7. b
8. b
9. a
10. a
11. b
12. b

Chapter 15

1. b
2. c
3. b
4. d
5. c
6. b
7. b
8. a

9. a
10. a
11. b
12. b

CHAPTER 16

1. b
2. c
3. a
4. d
5. b
6. c
7. c
8. a
9. b
10. b
11. d
12. c

CHAPTER 17

1. a
2. c
3. b
4. b
5. a
6. c
7. a
8. c
9. d
10. c
11. c
12. a
13. a
14. b
15. d
16. d
17. d
18. a
19. a

20. c
21. c
22. d
23. a
24. d
25. d
26. a
27. d
28. a
29. b
30. c
31. c
32. c
33. d
34. a
35. a
36. d
37. b
38. a
39. c
40. d
41. d
42. d
43. d
44. b
45. c
46. a
47. a
48. a
49. d
50. a
51. d
52. a
53. a
54. a
55. c
56. a
57. b
58. c
59. b

60. c
61. c
62. c
63. a
64. a
65. b
66. c
67. d
68. c
69. c
70. d
71. a
72. b
73. c
74. b
75. c
76. d
77. c
78. a
79. b
80. a
81. c
82. c
83. a
84. a
85. b
86. a
87. a
88. a
89. c
90. b
91. d
92. a
93. d
94. a
95. b
96. a
97. b
98. a
99. a

100. b
101. b
102. c
103. a
104. d
105. c
106. a
107. a
108. a
109. b
110. b
111. c
112. a
113. a
114. c
115. b
116. a
117. c
118. a
119. b
120. c
121. a
122. d
123. c
124. d
125. a
126. b
127. d
128. c
129. b
130. b
131. a
132. b
133. c
134. d
135. c
136. a
137. b
138. d
139. c

140. a

141. d

142. b

143. b

144. b

145. b

146. c

147. b

148. b

149. a

150. c

APPENDIX 2

ANSWERS TO REVIEW STRIPS

CHAPTER 18
12-LEAD EKG REVIEW STRIPS

1. Rate: 66
   Rhythm: Regular
   P wave: Present, upright (II)
   PR Interval: 0.18 sec
   QRS complex: 0.08 sec
   ST elevation: V_1, V_2, V_3, V_4 with inversion of T wave
   ST depression: None
   Pathologic Q waves: None
   Interpretation: Normal sinus rhythm with anterior/lateral MI

2. Rate: 107
   Rhythm: Irregular
   P wave: Present, upright (II)
   PR Interval: 0.16 sec
   QRS complex: 0.13 sec
   ST elevation: II, III, aVF
   ST depression: None
   Pathologic Q waves: None
   Interpretation: Sinus tachycardia with frequent PVCs, inferior injury

3. Rate: 88
   Rhythm: Regular
   P wave: Present, notched (II)
   PR Interval: 0.20 sec
   QRS complex: 0.12 sec
   ST elevation: None
   ST depression: None

Pathologic Q waves: None
Interpretation: Normal sinus rhythm, left axis deviation, left bundle branch block

4. Rate: 74
    Rhythm: Regular
    P wave: Inverted (III)
    PR Interval: 0.20 sec
    QRS complex: 0.14 sec
    ST elevation: None
    ST depression: I, aVL
    Pathologic Q waves: II, III, aVF
    Interpretation: Junctional rhythm, inferior infarct, anterior ischemia

5. Rate: 55
    Rhythm: Irregular
    P wave: None present
    PR Interval: 0
    QRS complex: 0.16 sec
    ST elevation: None
    ST depression: None
    Pathologic Q waves: None
    Interpretation: Atrial fibrillation with junctional escape, right bundle branch block

6. Rate: 93
    Rhythm: Regular
    P wave: Present, upright (II)
    PR Interval: 0.15 sec
    QRS complex: 0.13 sec
    ST elevation: II, III, aVF
    ST depression: V_5, V_6
    Pathologic Q waves: II, aVF
    Interpretation: Normal sinus rhythm, inferior infarct, lateral ischemia, incomplete bundle branch block

7. Rate: 73
    Rhythm: Regular
    P wave: Present, notched (II)
    PR Interval: 0.14 sec
    QRS complex: 0.08 sec
    ST elevation: None
    ST depression: None
    Pathologic Q waves: None
    Interpretation: Normal sinus rhythm, left axis deviation

8. Rate: 99
   Rhythm: Irregular
   P wave: Present, upright (II)
   PR Interval: 0.14 sec
   QRS complex: 0.08 sec
   ST elevation: II, III, aVF
   ST depression: None
   Pathologic Q waves: II, III, aVF
   Interpretation: Normal sinus rhythm with sinus dysrhythmia, inferior infarct pattern

9. Rate: 200
   Rhythm: Regular
   P wave: Not present
   PR Interval: 0
   QRS complex: 0.07 sec
   ST elevation: None
   ST depression: None
   Pathologic Q waves: None
   Interpretation: Supraventricular tachycardia

10. Rate: 60
    Rhythm: Regular
    P wave: Present, upright (II)
    PR Interval: 0.17 sec
    QRS complex: 0.10 sec
    ST elevation: V_1, V_2, V_3, V_4 with T wave inversion
    ST depression: None
    Pathologic Q waves: None
    Interpretation: Normal sinus rhythm, anterior/lateral injury

11. Rate: 68
    Rhythm: Regular
    P wave: Present (II)
    PR Interval: 0.12 sec
    QRS complex: 0.06 sec
    ST elevation: II, III, aVF, V_5, V_6
    ST depression: None
    Pathologic Q waves: None
    Interpretation: Normal sinus rhythm, inferolateral infarct

12. Rate: 94
    Rhythm: Regular
    P wave: Present (II)

PR Interval:	0.12 sec
QRS complex:	0.08 sec
ST elevation:	II, III, aVF
ST depression:	V_1, V_2, V_3, V_4
Pathologic Q waves:	None
Interpretation:	Normal sinus rhythm, acute inferior infarct

13. Rate: 75

Rhythm:	Regular
P wave:	Present, notched (II)
PR Interval:	0.20 sec
QRS complex:	0.08 sec
ST elevation:	V_1, V_2, V_3, V_4, V_5, V_6
ST depression:	None
Pathologic Q waves:	None
Interpretation:	Normal sinus rhythm, anterolateral infarct pattern

14. Rate: >200

Rhythm:	Irregular
P wave:	None present
PR Interval:	0
QRS complex:	0.16 sec
ST elevation:	None
ST depression:	None
Pathologic Q waves:	None
Interpretation:	Ventricular tachycardia

15. Rate: 78

Rhythm:	Regular
P wave:	Present
PR Interval:	0.12 sec
QRS complex:	0.08 sec
ST elevation:	Slight in II, III, aVF with T wave inversion
ST depression:	None
Pathologic Q waves:	None
Interpretation:	Normal sinus rhythm, inferior ischemia

16. Rate: 74

Rhythm:	Regular
P wave:	Present
PR Interval:	0.22 sec
QRS complex:	0.08 sec
ST elevation:	V_1, V_2, V_3, V_4 with poor R wave progression

ST depression: None

Pathologic Q waves: None

Interpretation: Sinus rhythm with first-degree block, anteroseptal infarct

17. Rate: 60

    Rhythm: Regular

    P wave: Present

    PR Interval: 0.26 sec

    QRS complex: 0.08 sec

    ST elevation: None

    ST depression: None

    Pathologic Q waves: None

    Interpretation: Normal sinus rhythm with first-degree block

18. Rate: 74

    Rhythm: Regular

    P wave: Present, upright (II)

    PR Interval: 0.18 sec

    QRS complex: 0.08 sec

    ST elevation: V_1, V_2, V_3, V_4 with T wave inversion

    ST depression: None

    Pathologic Q waves: None

    Interpretation: Normal sinus rhythm, left axis deviation, anteroseptal infarct

19. Rate: 88

    Rhythm: Regular

    P wave: Present, upright (II)

    PR Interval: 0.14 sec

    QRS complex: 0.08 sec

    ST elevation: II, III, aVF

    ST depression: I, aVL

    Pathologic Q waves: None

    Interpretation: Normal sinus rhythm, right axis deviation, inferior infarct

20. Rate: 87

    Rhythm: Regular

    P wave: Present, upright (II)

    PR Interval: 0.16 sec

    QRS complex: 0.08 sec

    ST elevation: V_1, V_2, V_3, V_4, V_5, V_6

    ST depression: None

    Pathologic Q waves: None

    Interpretation: Normal sinus rhythm, anterolateral infarct

21. Rate: 71
    Rhythm: Regular
    P wave: None
    PR Interval: 0
    QRS complex: 0.14 sec
    ST elevation: None
    ST depression: None
    Pathologic Q waves: None
    Interpretation: Pacer rhythm

22. Rate: 74
    Rhythm: Regular
    P wave: Present, upright (II)
    PR Interval: 0.16 sec
    QRS complex: 0.08 sec
    ST elevation: I, aVL, V_2, V_3, V_4, V_5, V_6
    ST depression: III, aVF
    Pathologic Q waves: None
    Interpretation: Normal sinus rhythm, anterolateral infarct

23. Rate: 98
    Rhythm: Regular
    P wave: None
    PR Interval: 0
    QRS complex: 0.12 sec
    ST elevation: I, II, III, aVL, aVF, V_1, V_2, V_3, V_4, V_5, V_6
    ST depression: aVR
    Pathologic Q waves: None
    Interpretation: Junctional rhythm with bigeminy PVCs, anteroseptal, inferolateral infarct

24. Rate: 68
    Rhythm: Regular
    P wave: Present, upright (II)
    PR Interval: 0.11 sec
    QRS complex: 0.04 sec
    ST elevation: None
    ST depression: None
    Pathologic Q waves: None
    Interpretation: Normal sinus rhythm

25. Rate: 67
    Rhythm: Irregular
    P wave: Present, upright (II)

PR Interval:	0.16 sec
QRS complex:	0.06 sec
ST elevation:	I, aVL, V_1, V_2, V_3, V_4
ST depression:	III, aVF
Pathologic Q waves:	None
Interpretation:	Normal sinus rhythm with sinus dysrhythmia, anteroseptal infarct

26. Rate: 108

Rhythm:	Irregular
P wave:	None
PR Interval:	0
QRS complex:	0.08 sec
ST elevation:	None
ST depression:	V_2, V_3, V_4
Pathologic Q waves:	III, aVF
Interpretation:	Atrial fibrillation with rapid ventricular response, inferior MI

27. Rate: 104

Rhythm:	Irregular
P wave:	Present, upright (II)
PR Interval:	0.12 sec
QRS complex:	0.08 sec
ST elevation:	None
ST depression:	None
Pathologic Q waves:	None
Interpretation:	Normal sinus rhythm with bigeminy PVCs

28. Rate: 55

Rhythm:	Regular
P wave:	Present, upright (II)
PR Interval:	0.10 sec
QRS complex:	0.08 sec
ST elevation:	None
ST depression:	None
Pathologic Q waves:	None
Interpretation:	Sinus bradycardia

29. Rate: 96

Rhythm:	Regular
P wave:	Present, upright (II)
PR Interval:	0.14 sec
QRS complex:	0.08 sec
ST elevation:	II, III, aVF, V_1, V_2, V_3

ST depression:	I, aVL
Pathologic Q waves:	III, aVF
Interpretation:	Normal sinus rhythm, inferior-anterior MI

30.
Rate:	79
Rhythm:	Regular
P wave:	Present, upright (II)
PR Interval:	0.16 sec
QRS complex:	0.08 sec
ST elevation:	I, aVL, V_1, V_2, V_3, V_4, V_5
ST depression:	None
Pathologic Q waves:	None
Interpretation:	Normal sinus rhythm, anterior MI

31.
Rate:	70
Rhythm:	Regular
P wave:	None
PR Interval:	0
QRS complex:	0.18 sec
ST elevation:	None
ST depression:	None
Pathologic Q waves:	None
Interpretation:	Pacer rhythm

32.
Rate:	90
Rhythm:	Irregular
P wave:	Present, upright (II)
PR Interval:	0.16 sec
QRS complex:	0.12 sec
ST elevation:	None
ST depression:	II, III, aVF
Pathologic Q waves:	None
Interpretation:	Normal sinus rhythm going into V-tach/V-fib with inferior ischemia

33.
Rate:	50
Rhythm:	Regular
P wave:	Present, upright (II)
PR Interval:	0.32 sec
QRS complex:	0.12 sec
ST elevation:	II, III, aVF
ST depression:	I, aVL, V_2, V_3
Pathologic Q waves:	None
Interpretation:	Second-degree block Type II, inferior MI, posterior MI

34. Rate: 69

Rhythm:	Regular
P wave:	Present, upright (II); delta waves
PR Interval:	0.08 sec
QRS complex:	0.08 sec
ST elevation:	None
ST depression:	None
Pathologic Q waves:	None
Interpretation:	Normal sinus rhythm with sinus dysrhythmia, Wolff-Parkinson-White syndrome

35. Rate: 55

Rhythm:	Regular
P wave:	Present, upright (II)
PR Interval:	0.22 sec
QRS complex:	0.08 sec
ST elevation:	II, III, aVF
ST depression:	I, aVL, V_1, V_2, V_3, V_4
Pathologic Q waves:	None
Interpretation:	Sinus bradycardia with first-degree block, inferior MI

36. Rate: 57

Rhythm:	Irregular
P wave:	None
PR Interval:	0
QRS complex:	0.08 sec
ST elevation:	V_5, V_6
ST depression:	None
Pathologic Q waves:	None
Interpretation:	Atrial flutter, lateral infarct

37. Rate: 99

Rhythm:	Regular
P wave:	Present, upright (II)
PR Interval:	0.17 sec
QRS complex:	0.08 sec
ST elevation:	II, aVF
ST depression:	I, aVL, V_2, V_3
Pathologic Q waves:	III, aVF
Interpretation:	Normal sinus rhythm, inferior MI, anterior ischemia

38. Rate: 70

Rhythm:	Regular

P wave:	Present (II)
PR Interval:	0.12 sec
QRS complex:	0.08 sec
ST elevation:	I, II, III, aVL, V_3, V_4, V_5, V_6
ST depression:	None
Pathologic Q waves:	None
Interpretation:	Normal sinus rhythm, anterior/inferolateral MI

39. Rate: 64

Rhythm:	Regular
P wave:	Present, notched (II)
PR Interval:	0.20 sec
QRS complex:	0.12 sec
ST elevation:	II, III, aVF
ST depression:	aVR, aVL, V_1, V_2, V_3
Pathologic Q waves:	None
Interpretation:	Normal sinus rhythm, inferior MI, septal ischemia

40. Rate: 55

Rhythm:	Regular
P wave:	Present, upright (II)
PR Interval:	0.16 sec
QRS complex:	0.08 sec
ST elevation:	V_1, V_2, V_3, V_4, V_5, V_6 with T wave inversion
ST depression:	None
Pathologic Q waves:	None
Interpretation:	Sinus bradycardia, anterolateral MI

41. Rate: 50

Rhythm:	Regular
P wave:	Present, upright (II)
PR Interval:	Variable
QRS complex:	0.10 sec
ST elevation:	II, III, aVF, V_5, V_6
ST depression:	I, aVL, V_1, V_2
Pathologic Q waves:	None
Interpretation:	Third-degree block, right axis deviation, inferolateral MI

42. Rate: 88

Rhythm:	Regular
P wave:	Present, upright (II)
PR Interval:	0.16 sec
QRS complex:	0.10 sec

ST elevation:	I, II, III, aVF, V_1, V_2, V_3, V_4, V_5, V_6
ST depression:	None
Pathologic Q waves:	None
Interpretation:	Normal sinus rhythm, anterolateral MI, inferior MI

43. Rate: 67

Rhythm:	Regular
P wave:	Present, upright (II)
PR Interval:	0.12 sec
QRS complex:	0.08 sec
ST elevation:	I, aVL, V_1, V_2, V_3, V_4
ST depression:	II, III, aVF
Pathologic Q waves:	None
Interpretation:	Normal sinus rhythm, anteroseptal MI

44. Rate: 70

Rhythm:	Regular
P wave:	Present, upright (II)
PR Interval:	0.16 sec
QRS complex:	0.08 sec
ST elevation:	V_1, V_2, V_3, V_4, V_5, V_6 with T wave inversion
ST depression:	None
Pathologic Q waves:	None
Interpretation:	Normal sinus rhythm, anterolateral MI

45. Rate: 82

Rhythm:	Regular
P wave:	Present, upright (II)
PR Interval:	0.16 sec
QRS complex:	0.08 sec
ST elevation:	None
ST depression:	None
Pathologic Q waves:	None
Interpretation:	Normal sinus rhythm

46. Rate: 69

Rhythm:	Regular
P wave:	Present, notched (II)
PR Interval:	0.24 sec
QRS complex:	0.08 sec
ST elevation:	None
ST depression:	None
Pathologic Q waves:	None
Interpretation:	Normal sinus rhythm with first-degree block

47. Rate: 75

    Rhythm: Regular

    P wave: Present, notched (II)

    PR Interval: 0.16 sec

    QRS complex: 0.08 sec

    ST elevation: Slight in I, aVL, V_1, V_2, V_3, V_4, V_5 with T wave inversion

    ST depression: None

    Pathologic Q waves: None

    Interpretation: Normal sinus rhythm, left axis deviation, anterolateral ischemia

48. Rate: 79

    Rhythm: Regular

    P wave: Present, upright (II)

    PR Interval: 0.18 sec

    QRS complex: 0.08 sec

    ST elevation: II, III, aVF

    ST depression: I, aVL, V_1, V_2, V_3, V_4, V_5

    Pathologic Q waves: II, III, aVF

    Interpretation: Normal sinus rhythm, inferior MI

49. Rate: 74

    Rhythm: Regular

    P wave: Present, upright (II)

    PR Interval: 0.20 sec

    QRS complex: 0.08 sec

    ST elevation: V_1, V_2, V_3, V_4

    ST depression: None

    Pathologic Q waves: None

    Interpretation: Normal sinus rhythm, anteroseptal MI

50. Rate: 71

    Rhythm: Irregular

    P wave: Present, upright (II)

    PR Interval: Varies

    QRS complex: 0.08 sec

    ST elevation: None

    ST depression: None

    Pathologic Q waves: II, aVF

    Interpretation: Normal sinus rhythm with second-degree block Mobitz Type I, left axis deviation, consider old inferior MI

51. Rate: 150

    Rhythm: Regular

P wave:	If present, hidden in QRS complex
PR Interval:	0
QRS complex:	0.16 sec
ST elevation:	I, aVL, V$_1$, V$_2$, V$_3$, V$_4$, V$_5$, V$_6$
ST depression:	None
Pathologic Q waves:	None
Interpretation:	Wide complex tachycardia, left axis deviation, anterolateral/septal MI

52.	Rate:	90
	Rhythm:	Irregular
	P wave:	Absent
	PR Interval:	0
	QRS complex:	0.08 sec
	ST elevation:	None
	ST depression:	None
	Pathologic Q waves:	None
	Interpretation:	Accelerated junctional rhythm with bigeminy PVCs and couplet PVCs

53.	Rate:	84
	Rhythm:	Regular
	P wave:	Present, upright (II)
	PR Interval:	0.16 sec
	QRS complex:	0.08 sec
	ST elevation:	II, III, aVF
	ST depression:	I, aVL, V$_2$, V$_3$, V$_4$, V$_5$
	Pathologic Q waves:	None
	Interpretation:	Normal sinus rhythm, inferior MI

54.	Rate:	138
	Rhythm:	Regular
	P wave:	Absent or hidden in QRS complex
	PR Interval:	0
	QRS complex:	0.16 sec
	ST elevation:	I, aVL, V$_1$, V$_2$, V$_3$, V$_4$, V$_5$, V$_6$
	ST depression:	None
	Pathologic Q waves:	None
	Interpretation:	Wide complex tachycardia, anteroseptal-lateral MI

55.	Rate:	128
	Rhythm:	Regular
	P wave:	Present, upright (II)
	PR Interval:	0.16 sec
	QRS complex:	0.08 sec

ST elevation:	None
ST depression:	V_4, V_5, V_6
Pathologic Q waves:	None
Interpretation:	Normal sinus rhythm, lateral ischemia

56. Rate: 121
Rhythm:	Regular
P wave:	Present, upright (II)
PR Interval:	0.16 sec
QRS complex:	0.08 sec
ST elevation:	None
ST depression:	None
Pathologic Q waves:	None
Interpretation:	Sinus tachycardia

57. Rate: 35
Rhythm:	Irregular
P wave:	Absent
PR Interval:	0
QRS complex:	0.08 sec
ST elevation:	None
ST depression:	V_2, V_3, V_4, V_5, V_6
Pathologic Q waves:	None
Interpretation:	Junctional bradycardia with PJCs, anterolateral ischemia

58. Rate: 124
Rhythm:	Regular
P wave:	Present, upright (II)
PR Interval:	0.18 sec
QRS complex:	0.08 sec
ST elevation:	V_1, V_2
ST depression:	None
Pathologic Q waves:	None
Interpretation:	Sinus tachycardia, septal MI

59. Rate: 96
Rhythm:	Regular
P wave:	Present, upright (II)
PR Interval:	0.16 sec
QRS complex:	0.12 sec
ST elevation:	None
ST depression:	None
Pathologic Q waves:	None
Interpretation:	Normal sinus rhythm, left bundle branch block

60. Rate: 59
    Rhythm: Regular
    P wave: Absent
    PR Interval: 0
    QRS complex: 0.14 sec
    ST elevation: None
    ST depression: None
    Pathologic Q waves: None
    Interpretation: Ventricular pacemaker rhythm

61. Rate: 70
    Rhythm: Regular
    P wave: Flutter waves
    PR Interval: 0
    QRS complex: 0.08 sec
    ST elevation: None
    ST depression: None
    Pathologic Q waves: None
    Interpretation: Atrial flutter

62. Rate: 68
    Rhythm: Irregular
    P wave: Present, upright (II)
    PR Interval: 0.12 sec
    QRS complex: 0.08 sec
    ST elevation: II, III, aVF
    ST depression: I, aVL, V_3, V_4, V_5, V_6
    Pathologic Q waves: II, aVF
    Interpretation: Sinus dysrhythmia, inferior MI

63. Rate: 96
    Rhythm: Regular
    P wave: Present, upright (II)
    PR Interval: 0.12 sec
    QRS complex: 0.08 sec
    ST elevation: II, III, aVF, V_2, V_3, V_4
    ST depression: None
    Pathologic Q waves: None
    Interpretation: Normal sinus rhythm, inferior/anterior MI

64. Rate: 86
    Rhythm: Irregular
    P wave: Absent

PR Interval:	0
QRS complex:	0.04 sec
ST elevation:	None
ST depression:	None
Pathologic Q waves:	None
Interpretation:	Junctional rhythm with run of V-tach

65. | Rate: | 43 |
Rhythm:	Regular
P wave:	Present, upright (II)
PR Interval:	0.22 sec
QRS complex:	0.08 sec
ST elevation:	II, III, aVF, V_3, V_4, V_5, V_6
ST depression:	I, aVL, V_1, V_2
Pathologic Q waves:	None
Interpretation:	Second-degree block Type II, anterior/inferolateral MI, right axis deviation

66. | Rate: | 88 |
Rhythm:	Regular
P wave:	Present, upright (II)
PR Interval:	0.16 sec
QRS complex:	0.08 sec
ST elevation:	I, aVL, V_1, V_2, V_3, V_4, V_5, V_6
ST depression:	III, aVR
Pathologic Q waves:	None
Interpretation:	Normal sinus rhythm, anterolateral MI

67. | Rate: | 67 |
Rhythm:	Regular
P wave:	Present, upright (II)
PR Interval:	0.12 sec
QRS complex:	0.04 sec
ST elevation:	I, aVL, V_1, V_2, V_3, V_4 (tombstones)
ST depression:	II, III, aVF
Pathologic Q waves:	None
Interpretation:	Normal sinus rhythm, anteroseptal MI

68. | Rate: | 96 |
Rhythm:	Irregular
P wave:	Present, notched (II)
PR Interval:	0.32 sec
QRS complex:	0.11 sec

ST elevation:	I, II, III, aVL, aVF, V_1, V_2, V_3, V_4, V_5, V_6
ST depression:	None
Pathologic Q waves:	None
Interpretation:	Sinus rhythm with first-degree block and run of bigeminy PVCs, anteroseptal MI, inferolateral MI

69. Rate: 85

Rhythm:	Regular
P wave:	Present, upright (II)
PR Interval:	0.16 sec
QRS complex:	0.04 sec
ST elevation:	II, III, aVF
ST depression:	None
Pathologic Q waves:	III, aVF
Interpretation:	Normal sinus rhythm, inferior MI

70. Rate: 117

Rhythm:	Regular
P wave:	Present, upright (II)
PR Interval:	0.16 sec
QRS complex:	0.04 sec
ST elevation:	None
ST depression:	None
Pathologic Q waves:	None
Interpretation:	Sinus tachycardia rhythm

71. Rate: 146

Rhythm:	Regular
P wave:	Absent
PR Interval:	0
QRS complex:	0.12 sec
ST elevation:	None
ST depression:	V_4, V_5, V_6
Pathologic Q waves:	None
Interpretation:	Supraventricular rhythm with run of V-tach, lateral ischemia

72. Rate: 115

Rhythm:	Regular
P wave:	Present, upright (II)
PR Interval:	0.16 sec
QRS complex:	0.08 sec
ST elevation:	II, III, aVF
ST depression:	I, aVL, V_1, V_2, V_3, V_4, V_5, V_6

Pathologic Q waves: III, aVF

Interpretation: Sinus tachycardia, inferior MI, anterior ischemia

73. Rate: 74

Rhythm: Regular

P wave: Present, upright (II)

PR Interval: 0.16 sec

QRS complex: 0.08 sec

ST elevation: II, III, aVF

ST depression: I, aVL

Pathologic Q waves: None

Interpretation: Normal sinus rhythm, inferior MI

74. Rate: 93

Rhythm: Irregular

P wave: Present, upright (II)

PR Interval: 0.16 sec

QRS complex: 0.08 sec

ST elevation: None

ST depression: V_4, V_5, V_6

Pathologic Q waves: None

Interpretation: Normal sinus rhythm with PJCs, lateral ischemia

75. Rate: 128

Rhythm: Regular

P wave: Absent

PR Interval: 0

QRS complex: 0.10 sec

ST elevation: II, III, aVF

ST depression: None

Pathologic Q waves: None

Interpretation: Supraventricular tachycardia, left axis deviation, right bundle branch block, inferior MI

76. Rate: 88

Rhythm: Irregular

P wave: Present, upright (II)

PR Interval: 0.16 sec

QRS complex: 0.08 sec

ST elevation: None

ST depression: None

Pathologic Q waves: Poor R wave progression, V_1, V_2, V_3

Interpretation: Sinus rhythm with occasional PACs, consider old septal MI

77. Rate: 123
    Rhythm: Irregular
    P wave: Absent
    PR Interval: 0
    QRS complex: 0.10 sec
    ST elevation: None
    ST depression: None
    Pathologic Q waves: II, III, aVF
    Interpretation: Atrial fibrillation with rapid ventricular response, left axis deviation, left bundle branch block, consider inferior MI (old), right bundle branch block, demand pacemaker firing twice

78. Rate: 86
    Rhythm: Regular
    P wave: Present, upright (II)
    PR Interval: 0.16 sec
    QRS complex: 0.08 sec
    ST elevation: II, aVF, V_2, V_3, V_4
    ST depression: I, aVL
    Pathologic Q waves: III, aVF
    Interpretation: Normal sinus rhythm, inferior MI, anterior MI

79. Rate: 70
    Rhythm: Regular
    P wave: Present, upright (II)
    PR Interval: 0.16 sec
    QRS complex: 0.06 sec
    ST elevation: II, III, aVF, V_5, V_6
    ST depression: None
    Pathologic Q waves: None
    Interpretation: Normal sinus rhythm, inferolateral MI

80. Rate: 64
    Rhythm: Irregular
    P wave: Present, upright (II)
    PR Interval: 0.14 sec
    QRS complex: 0.12 sec
    ST elevation: None
    ST depression: None
    Pathologic Q waves: None
    Interpretation: Sinus rhythm with premature ventricular complexes

81. Rate: 86
    Rhythm: Regular

P wave:	Present, upright (II)
PR Interval:	0.16 sec
QRS complex:	0.08 sec
ST elevation:	II, III, aVF
ST depression:	aVL, V_1, V_2, V_3, V_4
Pathologic Q waves:	None
Interpretation:	Normal sinus rhythm, inferior MI

82.
Rate:	60
Rhythm:	Regular
P wave:	Present, upright (II)
PR Interval:	0.18 sec
QRS complex:	0.08 sec
ST elevation:	V_1, V_2, V_3, V_4, V_5, with T wave inversion
ST depression:	T wave inversion in I, aVL
Pathologic Q waves:	None
Interpretation:	Normal sinus rhythm, anterolateral MI

83.
Rate:	72
Rhythm:	Irregular
P wave:	Present, upright (II)
PR Interval:	0.18 sec
QRS complex:	0.14 sec
ST elevation:	None
ST depression:	None
Pathologic Q waves:	None
Interpretation:	Sinus rhythm with occasional PVCs, left axis deviation, left bundle branch block

84.
Rate:	74
Rhythm:	Irregular
P wave:	Absent
PR Interval:	0
QRS complex:	0.14 sec
ST elevation:	II, III, aVF
ST depression:	None
Pathologic Q waves:	None
Interpretation:	Junctional rhythm with PJCs, right bundle branch block, inferior MI

85.
Rate:	80
Rhythm:	Regular
P wave:	Present, upright (II)
PR Interval:	0.16 sec

QRS complex:	0.08 sec
ST elevation:	II, III, aVF
ST depression:	None
Pathologic Q waves:	III, aVF
Interpretation:	Normal sinus rhythm, incomplete right bundle branch block, inferior MI

86. Rate: 98

Rhythm:	Regular
P wave:	Present, upright (II)
PR Interval:	0.16 sec
QRS complex:	0.08 sec
ST elevation:	I, aVL, V_2, V_3, V_4, V_5, V_6
ST depression:	None
Pathologic Q waves:	None
Interpretation:	Normal sinus rhythm, anterolateral MI

87. Rate: 130

Rhythm:	Irregular
P wave:	Absent
PR Interval:	0
QRS complex:	0.06 sec
ST elevation:	None
ST depression:	None
Pathologic Q waves:	Poor R wave progression
Interpretation:	Atrial fibrillation with rapid ventricular response, consider anteroseptal injury

88. Rate: 118

Rhythm:	Irregular
P wave:	Absent
PR Interval:	0
QRS complex:	0.08 sec
ST elevation:	None
ST depression:	None
Pathologic Q waves:	Poor R wave progression
Interpretation:	Atrial fibrillation with rapid ventricular response

89. Rate: 84

Rhythm:	Regular
P wave:	Present, upright (II)
PR Interval:	0.16 sec
QRS complex:	0.04 sec
ST elevation:	V_5, V_6

ST depression:	aVR, V_1, V_2, V_3
Pathologic Q waves:	None
Interpretation:	Normal sinus rhythm, lateral MI

90. | | |
|---|---|
| Rate: | 88 |
| Rhythm: | Regular |
| P wave: | Present, upright (II) |
| PR Interval: | 0.14 sec |
| QRS complex: | 0.08 sec |
| ST elevation: | II, III, aVF |
| ST depression: | I, aVR, aVL |
| Pathologic Q waves: | None |
| Interpretation: | Normal sinus rhythm, right axis deviation, inferior MI |

91. | | |
|---|---|
| Rate: | 68 |
| Rhythm: | Irregular |
| P wave: | Present, upright (II) |
| PR Interval: | 0.12 sec |
| QRS complex: | 0.06 sec |
| ST elevation: | I, aVL, V_2, V_3, V_4, V_5, V_6 |
| ST depression: | None |
| Pathologic Q waves: | None |
| Interpretation: | Sinus rhythm with occasional PVCs, anterior/lateral MI |

92. | | |
|---|---|
| Rate: | 80 |
| Rhythm: | Iregular |
| P wave: | Present, upright (II) |
| PR Interval: | 0.12 sec |
| QRS complex: | 0.6 sec |
| ST elevation: | I, aVL, V_1, V_2, V_3, V_4, V_5, V_6 |
| ST depression: | II, III, aVF |
| Pathologic Q waves: | None |
| Interpretation: | Sinus rhythm with occasional PVCs, anterolateral MI |

93. | | |
|---|---|
| Rate: | 92 |
| Rhythm: | Irregular |
| P wave: | Present, upright (II) |
| PR Interval: | 0.22 sec |
| QRS complex: | 0.08 sec |
| ST elevation: | None |
| ST depression: | None |
| Pathologic Q waves: | Poor R wave progression |
| Interpretation: | Sinus rhythm with first-degree block with PVCs |

94. Rate: 69

     Rhythm: Regular

     P wave: Present, upright (II)

     PR Interval: 0.08 sec

     QRS complex: 0.11 sec

     ST elevation: None

     ST depression: None

     Pathologic Q waves: None

     Interpretation: Normal sinus rhythm with sinus dysrhythmia, Wolff-Parkinson-White syndrome (delta waves)

95. Rate: 74

     Rhythm: Irregular

     P wave: Present, upright (II)

     PR Interval: 0.16 sec

     QRS complex: 0.08 sec

     ST elevation: I, aVL, V_1, V_2, V_3, V_4

     ST depression: V_5, V_6

     Pathologic Q waves: None

     Interpretation: Sinus rhythm with frequent PVCs, anteroseptal MI, lateral ischemia

96. Rate: 67

     Rhythm: Regular

     P wave: Present, upright (II)

     PR Interval: 0.16 sec

     QRS complex: 0.08 sec

     ST elevation: I, aVL, V_1, V_2, V_3, V_4

     ST depression: II, III, aVF

     Pathologic Q waves: None

     Interpretation: Normal sinus rhythm, anterior MI (tombstones)

97. Rate: 128

     Rhythm: Irregular

     P wave: Present, upright (II)

     PR Interval: 0.16 sec

     QRS complex: 0.06 sec

     ST elevation: V_1, V_2, V_3, V_4, V_5

     ST depression: None

     Pathologic Q waves: Poor R wave progression

     Interpretation: Sinus tachycardia with occasional PJCs, consider anterior MI

98. Rate: 77

     Rhythm: Irregular

P wave:	Present, upright (II)
PR Interval:	0.16 sec
QRS complex:	0.08 sec
ST elevation:	I, aVL, V_1, V_2, V_3, V_4, V_5
ST depression:	II, aVF
Pathologic Q waves:	None
Interpretation:	Sinus rhythm with sinus dysrhythmia, anterolateral MI

99.
Rate:	38
Rhythm:	Regular
P wave:	Present
PR Interval:	Variable
QRS complex:	0.08 sec
ST elevation:	II, III, aVF, V_4, V_5, V_6
ST depression:	I, aVL, V_1, V_2, V_3
Pathologic Q waves:	None
Interpretation:	Third-degree block, right axis deviation, inferolateral MI

100.
Rate:	54
Rhythm:	Regular
P wave:	Present, upright (II)
PR Interval:	0.18 sec
QRS complex:	0.08 sec
ST elevation:	II, III, aVF
ST depression:	aVL, V_2
Pathologic Q waves:	None
Interpretation:	Sinus bradycardia, inferior MI

101.
Rate:	98
Rhythm:	Regular
P wave:	Present, upright (II)
PR Interval:	0.16 sec
QRS complex:	0.08 sec
ST elevation:	II, aVF
ST depression:	I, aVL, V_1, V_2, V_3
Pathologic Q waves:	None
Interpretation:	Normal sinus rhythm, inferior MI

102.
Rate:	60
Rhythm:	Regular
P wave:	Present, upright (II)
PR Interval:	0.16 sec
QRS complex:	0.08 sec

ST elevation:	I, aVL, V$_1$, V$_2$, V$_3$, V$_4$
ST depression:	None
Pathologic Q waves:	None
Interpretation:	Normal sinus rhythm, anterior MI, lateral ischemia (T wave inversion)

103. Rate: 88

Rhythm:	Regular
P wave:	Present, upright (II)
PR Interval:	0.16 sec
QRS complex:	0.06 sec
ST elevation:	None
ST depression:	None
Pathologic Q waves:	None
Interpretation:	Normal sinus rhythm

104. Rate: 62

Rhythm:	Irregular
P wave:	Present, upright (II)
PR Interval:	0.08 sec
QRS complex:	0.08 sec
ST elevation:	II, III, aVF
ST depression:	I, aVL, V$_2$, V$_3$, V$_4$, V$_5$
Pathologic Q waves:	II, III, aVF
Interpretation:	Sinus rhythm with sinus dysrhythmia with short PR Interval, inferior MI, consider also posterior MI

105. Rate: 44

Rhythm:	Regular
P wave:	Present, inverted (II)
PR Interval:	0.16 sec
QRS complex:	0.08 sec
ST elevation:	None
ST depression:	I, aVL, V$_1$, V$_2$, V$_3$, V$_4$, V$_5$, V$_6$
Pathologic Q waves:	None
Interpretation:	Junctional rhythm, septal MI (inverted T waves), lateral ischemia, right bundle branch block

106. Rate: 86

Rhythm:	Regular
P wave:	Present, upright (II)
PR Interval:	0.16 sec
QRS complex:	0.08 sec
ST elevation:	None

ST depression:	None
Pathologic Q waves:	None
Interpretation:	Normal sinus rhythm

107.
Rate:	88
Rhythm:	Regular
P wave:	Present, upright (II)
PR Interval:	0.16 sec
QRS complex:	0.08 sec
ST elevation:	I, II, III, aVF, V_1, V_2, V_3, V_4, V_5, V_6
ST depression:	None
Pathologic Q waves:	Poor R wave progression
Interpretation:	Normal sinus rhythm, anterolateral MI, inferior MI

108.
Rate:	78
Rhythm:	Regular
P wave:	Present, upright (II)
PR Interval:	0.12 sec
QRS complex:	0.08 sec
ST elevation:	I, aVL, V_2, V_3, V_4, V_5, V_6
ST depression:	III, aVF
Pathologic Q waves:	None
Interpretation:	Sinus rhythm with sinus dysrhythmia, anterolateral MI

109.
Rate:	74
Rhythm:	Regular
P wave:	Present, upright (II)
PR Interval:	0.16 sec
QRS complex:	0.08 sec
ST elevation:	I, aVL, V_1, V_2, V_3, V_4
ST depression:	III, aVF
Pathologic Q waves:	None
Interpretation:	Normal sinus rhythm, anterior MI

110.
Rate:	89
Rhythm:	Regular
P wave:	Present, upright (II)
PR Interval:	0.12 sec
QRS complex:	0.06 sec
ST elevation:	II, III, aVF
ST depression:	I, aVL, V_2, V_3
Pathologic Q waves:	None
Interpretation:	Normal sinus rhythm, right axis deviation, inferior MI

111. Rate: 112

      Rhythm: Regular

      P wave: Absent

      PR Interval: 0

      QRS complex: 0.18 sec

      ST elevation: None

      ST depression: None

      Pathologic Q waves: None

      Interpretation: AV sequential or dual-chamber electronic pacemaker

112. Rate: 55

      Rhythm: Regular

      P wave: Present, upright (II)

      PR Interval: 0.14 sec

      QRS complex: 0.06 sec

      ST elevation: V_1, V_2

      ST depression: None

      Pathologic Q waves: None

      Interpretation: Sinus bradycardia, consider septal MI

113. Rate: 69

      Rhythm: Irregular

      P wave: Present, upright (II)

      PR Interval: 0.12 sec

      QRS complex: 0.08 sec

      ST elevation: I, II, aVL, aVF, V_1, V_2, V_3, V_4, V_5, V_6

      ST depression: None

      Pathologic Q waves: None

      Interpretation: Sinus rhythm with occasional PVC, anterior MI, inferolateral MI

114. Rate: 62

      Rhythm: Regular

      P wave: Present, upright (II)

      PR Interval: 0.18 sec

      QRS complex: 0.08 sec

      ST elevation: None

      ST depression: V_1, V_2, V_3, V_4

      Pathologic Q waves: II, III, aVF

      Interpretation: Normal sinus rhythm, inferior MI (old), right bundle branch block

115. Rate: 79

      Rhythm: Regular

      P wave: Present, upright (II)

PR Interval:	0.12 sec
QRS complex:	0.11 sec
ST elevation:	II, III, aVF, V_5, V_6
ST depression:	I, aVL, V_1, V_2, V_3, V_4
Pathologic Q waves:	None
Interpretation:	Normal sinus rhythm, inferolateral MI

116. Rate: 62

Rhythm:	Regular
P wave:	Present, upright (II)
PR Interval:	0.22 sec
QRS complex:	0.08 sec
ST elevation:	II, III, aVF
ST depression:	I, aVL, V_1, V_2, V_3, V_4
Pathologic Q waves:	None
Interpretation:	Sinus rhythm with first-degree block, inferior MI

117. Rate: 77

Rhythm:	Regular
P wave:	Present, upright (II)
PR Interval:	0.16 sec
QRS complex:	0.12 sec
ST elevation:	V_1, V_2, V_3, V_4
ST depression:	II, III, aVF
Pathologic Q waves:	None
Interpretation:	Normal sinus rhythm, anteroseptal MI, right bundle branch block

118. Rate: 200

Rhythm:	Regular
P wave:	Absent or hidden
PR Interval:	0
QRS complex:	0.06 sec
ST elevation:	None
ST depression:	None
Pathologic Q waves:	None
Interpretation:	Supraventricular tachycardia

119. Rate: 86

Rhythm:	Regular
P wave:	Present, upright (II)
PR Interval:	0.16 sec
QRS complex:	0.08 sec
ST elevation:	II, III, aVF

ST depression:	I, aVL
Pathologic Q waves:	II, III, aVF
Interpretation:	Normal sinus rhythm, left axis deviation, inferior MI

120. | | |
|---|---|
| Rate: | 70 |
| Rhythm: | Regular |
| P wave: | Present, upright (II) |
| PR Interval: | 0.16 sec |
| QRS complex: | 0.08 sec |
| ST elevation: | None |
| ST depression: | I, aVL, V_2, V_3, V_4, V_5, V_6, T wave inversion in I, aVL, V_2, V_3, V_4, V_5, V_6 |
| Pathologic Q waves: | III, aVF |
| Interpretation: | Normal sinus rhythm, left axis deviation, inferior MI, anterolateral ischemia |

121. | | |
|---|---|
| Rate: | 76 |
| Rhythm: | Irregular |
| P wave: | Present, upright (II) |
| PR Interval: | 0.18 sec |
| QRS complex: | 0.08 sec |
| ST elevation: | V_1, V_2, V_3, V_4 |
| ST depression: | None |
| Pathologic Q waves: | None |
| Interpretation: | Sinus rhythm with frequent PJCs, anteroseptal MI, left axis deviation |

122. | | |
|---|---|
| Rate: | 66 |
| Rhythm: | Irregular |
| P wave: | Present, upright (II) |
| PR Interval: | 0.16 sec |
| QRS complex: | 0.08 sec |
| ST elevation: | V_1, V_2, V_3, V_4, V_5, V_6 |
| ST depression: | III, aVF |
| Pathologic Q waves: | None |
| Interpretation: | Sinus rhythm, anteroseptal MI |

123. | | |
|---|---|
| Rate: | 84 |
| Rhythm: | Regular |
| P wave: | Present, upright (II) |
| PR Interval: | 0.12 sec |
| QRS complex: | 0.04 sec |
| ST elevation: | None |
| ST depression: | None |
| Pathologic Q waves: | None |
| Interpretation: | Normal sinus rhythm |

124. Rate: 91
    Rhythm: Irregular
    P wave: Present, upright (II)
    PR Interval: 0.16 sec
    QRS complex: 0.08 sec
    ST elevation: None
    ST depression: V_1, V_2, V_3, V_4
    Pathologic Q waves: None
    Interpretation: Sinus rhythm with occasional PJCs, posterior MI (artifact)

125. Rate: 56
    Rhythm: Irregular
    P wave: Absent
    PR Interval: 0
    QRS complex: 0.08 sec
    ST elevation: I, II, aVF, aVL, V_2, V_3, V_4, V_5, V_6
    ST depression: None
    Pathologic Q waves: None
    Interpretation: Junctional rhythm with PVCs, anterior/inferolateral MI

126. Rate: 80
    Rhythm: Regular
    P wave: Present, upright (II)
    PR Interval: 0.12 sec
    QRS complex: 0.08 sec
    ST elevation: V_1, V_2, V_3, V_4
    ST depression: None
    Pathologic Q waves: II, III, aVF
    Interpretation: Normal sinus rhythm, anterior MI, inferior MI

127. Rate: 70
    Rhythm: Regular
    P wave: Present, upright (II)
    PR Interval: 0.16 sec
    QRS complex: 0.08 sec
    ST elevation: None
    ST depression: None
    Pathologic Q waves: None
    Interpretation: Normal sinus rhythm

128. Rate: 72
    Rhythm: Irregular
    P wave: Present, upright (II)

PR Interval:	0.12 sec
QRS complex:	0.08 sec
ST elevation:	I, aVL, V_1, V_2, V_3, V_4
ST depression:	II, III, aVF, V_5, V_6
Pathologic Q waves:	None
Interpretation:	Normal sinus rhythm with frequent PVCs, anteroseptal MI, lateral ischemia, left axis deviation

129. Rate: 60

Rhythm:	Regular
P wave:	Present, upright (II)
PR Interval:	0.12 sec
QRS complex:	0.06 sec
ST elevation:	I, aVL, V_1, V_2, V_3, V_4, V_5, V_6
ST depression:	III, aVF
Pathologic Q waves:	None
Interpretation:	Normal sinus rhythm, anteroseptal MI

130. Rate: 67

Rhythm:	Regular
P wave:	Present, upright (II)
PR Interval:	0.12 sec
QRS complex:	0.08 sec
ST elevation:	I, aVL, V_1, V_2, V_3, V_4
ST depression:	III, aVF
Pathologic Q waves:	None
Interpretation:	Normal sinus rhythm, anterior MI (tombstones in V_2, V_3)

131. Rate: 96

Rhythm:	Irregular
P wave:	Present, upright (II)
PR Interval:	0.28 sec
QRS complex:	0.10 sec
ST elevation:	I, II, III, aVL, aVF, V_1, V_2, V_3, V_4, V_5, V_6
ST depression:	None
Pathologic Q waves:	None
Interpretation:	Sinus rhythm with first-degree block, anteroseptal MI, inferolateral MI

132. Rate: 46

Rhythm:	Regular
P wave:	Present, upright (II)
PR Interval:	0.16 sec
QRS complex:	0.04 sec

ST elevation: V_1, V_2, V_3

ST depression: None

Pathologic Q waves: None

Interpretation: Sinus bradycardia rhythm, anterior MI

133. Rate: 78

     Rhythm: Regular

     P wave: Present, upright (II)

     PR Interval: 0.16 sec

     QRS complex: 0.08 sec

     ST elevation: None

     ST depression: None

     Pathologic Q waves: None

     Interpretation: Normal sinus rhythm

134. Rate: 46

     Rhythm: Regular

     P wave: Present, upright (II)

     PR Interval: 0.12 sec

     QRS complex: 0.08 sec

     ST elevation: II, III, aVF

     ST depression: None

     Pathologic Q waves: None

     Interpretation: Marked sinus bradycardia rhythm, inferior MI

135. Rate: 86

     Rhythm: Regular

     P wave: Present, upright (II)

     PR Interval: 0.16 sec

     QRS complex: 0.08 sec

     ST elevation: II, III, aVF, with T wave inversion

     ST depression: None

     Pathologic Q waves: II, III, aVF

     Interpretation: Normal sinus rhythm, inferior MI

136. Rate: 60

     Rhythm: Irregular

     P wave: Present, upright (II)

     PR Interval: 0.12 sec

     QRS complex: 0.10 sec

     ST elevation: V_1, V_2, V_3, V_4, V_5

     ST depression: None

     Pathologic Q waves: None

     Interpretation: Sinus rhythm with sinus dysrhythmia, anterolateral MI

137. Rate: 134
     Rhythm: Regular
     P wave: Present, upright (II)
     PR Interval: 0.16 sec
     QRS complex: 0.10 sec
     ST elevation: II, III, aVF
     ST depression: I, aVL, V_2, V_3, V_4, V_5, V_6
     Pathologic Q waves: None
     Interpretation: Sinus tachycardia rhythm, inferior-posterior MI

138. Rate: 75
     Rhythm: Regular
     P wave: Present, upright (II)
     PR Interval: 0.12 sec
     QRS complex: 0.08 sec
     ST elevation: None
     ST depression: III, aVF, V_2, V_3, V_4, V_5, V_6
     Pathologic Q waves: None
     Interpretation: Normal sinus rhythm, inferior/anterior ischemia

139. Rate: 78
     Rhythm: Irregular
     P wave: Absent
     PR Interval: 0
     QRS complex: 0.14 sec
     ST elevation: II, III, aVF
     ST depression: I, aVL, V_1, V_2, V_3, V_4
     Pathologic Q waves: None
     Interpretation: Atrial fibrillation, inferior MI, nonspecific intraventricular block

140. Rate: 110
     Rhythm: Regular
     P wave: Present, upright (II)
     PR Interval: 0.18 sec
     QRS complex: 0.08 sec
     ST elevation: None
     ST depression: I, aVL, V_3, V_4, V_5, V_6
     Pathologic Q waves: None
     Interpretation: Sinus tachycardia rhythm, consider anterolateral ischemia

141. Rate: 66
     Rhythm: Regular
     P wave: Present, upright (II)

PR Interval:	0.18 sec
QRS complex:	0.08 sec
ST elevation:	II, III, aVF
ST depression:	I, aVL, V_2, V_3
Pathologic Q waves:	None
Interpretation:	Normal sinus rhythm, inferior MI

142.
Rate:	70
Rhythm:	Regular
P wave:	Present, upright (II)
PR Interval:	0.16 sec
QRS complex:	0.08 sec
ST elevation:	I, II, aVL, aVF, V_3, V_4, V_5, V_6
ST depression:	aVR, V_1
Pathologic Q waves:	None
Interpretation:	Normal sinus rhythm, anterior MI, inferolateral MI

143.
Rate:	67
Rhythm:	Regular
P wave:	Present, upright (II)
PR Interval:	0.16 sec
QRS complex:	0.08 sec
ST elevation:	II, III, aVF
ST depression:	I, aVL, V_2, V_3, V_4, V_5
Pathologic Q waves:	None
Interpretation:	Normal sinus rhythm, inferior MI

144.
Rate:	80
Rhythm:	Regular
P wave:	Present, upright (II)
PR Interval:	0.12 sec
QRS complex:	0.12 sec
ST elevation:	I, aVL, V_1, V_2, V_3, V_4
ST depression:	None
Pathologic Q waves:	II, III, aVF
Interpretation:	Normal sinus rhythm, anteroseptal MI, inferior MI (old)

145.
Rate:	66
Rhythm:	Regular
P wave:	Present, inverted (II)
PR Interval:	0.16 sec
QRS complex:	0.08 sec
ST elevation:	II, III, aVF, V_5, V_6

ST depression:	V_1, V_2, V_3
Pathologic Q waves:	None
Interpretation:	Junctional rhythm, inferolateral MI

146. Rate: 74

Rhythm:	Irregular
P wave:	Present, upright (II)
PR Interval:	0.16 sec
QRS complex:	0.08 sec
ST elevation:	II, III, aVF, V_4, V_5, V_6
ST depression:	I, aVL, V_2, V_3
Pathologic Q waves:	None
Interpretation:	Sinus rhythm with trigeminy PVCs, inferolateral MI

147. Rate: 65

Rhythm:	Irregular
P wave:	Present, upright (II)
PR Interval:	0.16 sec
QRS complex:	0.08 sec
ST elevation:	I, II, III, aVF, aVL, V_2, V_3, V_4, V_5, V_6
ST depression:	aVR
Pathologic Q waves:	None
Interpretation:	Sinus rhythm with occasional PVCs, anterior MI, inferolateral MI

148. Rate: 72

Rhythm:	Irregular
P wave:	Present, upright (II)
PR Interval:	0.16 sec
QRS complex:	0.08 sec
ST elevation:	I, aVL, V_1, V_2, V_3
ST depression:	II, III, aVF, V_5, V_6
Pathologic Q waves:	None
Interpretation:	Sinus rhythm with frequent PVCs, anteroseptal MI, lateral ischemia

149. Rate: 38

Rhythm:	Regular
P wave:	Present, no relation with QRS complex
PR Interval:	variable
QRS complex:	0.12 sec
ST elevation:	II, III, aVF, V_2, V_3, V_4, V_5, V_6
ST depression:	None
Pathologic Q waves:	None
Interpretation:	Third-degree block, inferolateral MI, anterior MI, right bundle branch block

150. Rate: 112
    Rhythm: Regular
    P wave: Present, upright (II)
    PR Interval: 0.14 sec
    QRS complex: 0.08 sec
    ST elevation: III, aVF
    ST depression: V_3, V_4, V_5
    Pathologic Q waves: II, III, aVF
    Interpretation: Sinus tachycardia, inferior MI

151. Rate: 98
    Rhythm: Regular
    P wave: Present, upright (II)
    PR Interval: 0.16 sec
    QRS complex: 0.16 sec
    ST elevation: None
    ST depression: None
    Pathologic Q waves: None
    Interpretation: Normal sinus rhythm, left bundle branch block

152. Rate: 78
    Rhythm: Regular
    P wave: Present, upright (II)
    PR Interval: 0.16 sec
    QRS complex: 0.08 sec
    ST elevation: II, III, aVF
    ST depression: I, aVL, V_2, V_3, V_4, V_5
    Pathologic Q waves: III
    Interpretation: Normal sinus rhythm, inferior MI

INDEX

QRS complexes, 38–41
    analysis of, 53–54
    narrow, 54
    number of, 49–50
    pattern of, 51
    supraventricular, 54
    widening of, 54, 134–137
QRS mean axis, 131
qRS pattern, 136
QRS vector, 131
QS complexes indicating septal MIs, 104
Q waves, 39, 53
    absence of, 137
    as indication of subendocardial infarction,
        81–82
    as indication of transmural infarction, 81–82
    small, 136
    See also Pathologic Q waves

R

Receptors, adrenergic, 13–14, 160, 162–163, 165,
    169
Reciprocal changes, 83
Reciprocal leads, 83
    for detecting posterior MIs, 116–117, 121
Refractory period
    absolute and relative, 21
    prolonging, 168
    T wave representation of, 41
Relaxation, 17
Repolarization, 19–21, 41
    early, 56
    hypoxia effects on, 55
Resting membrane potential, 19
Resting phase, 41
    ion movement during, 19
    See also T waves
Retavase, 147–148
Rhythmicity, 17–18
Rhythm strips, 31
Right axis deviation, 132
Right bundle branch blocks (RBBB), 135–136,
    138–139
Right coronary artery, 63, 80–81, 91,
    117
    and inferior MIs, 80
Right ventricle
    delayed depolarization of, 135
    electrical supply to, 133
Right ventricular infarction (RVI), 85–86
R-R interval method, 50
rSR pattern, 136–137

R wave progression, 42
    absent, 94
    poor, 94, 104, 111
    and V lead analysis, 104
R waves, 39, 53
    counting number of, 50
    intervals between, 51
    narrow, 137
    notched, 137
    slurred, 137
    small, 137
    synchronizing electrical shocks with, 154
    tall, 121, 137

S

Scar tissue, 57
Semilunar valves, 5
Septal MIs, 100–101
    clinical significance of, 104–105
    EKG changes associated with, 104
    EKG strip example of, 102–104
    lead-specific changes indicating, 101–104
Septal perforating arteries, 101
Septum, 101
Sinoatrial (SA) node, 18, 25–26
    firing of, 38
    location of, 25
Sinus rhythm, 52
Sinus tachycardia, clinical significance of,
    96
6-second method, 49–50
Skin
    electrical impulses at, 31
    preparing for lead attachment, 35
Smooth muscle relaxants, 175–176
Sodium bicarbonate, 176–177
Sodium (Na) ions, 18–19
    movement into cells, 20
Sodium-potassium exchange pump, 19–20
Stacked shocks, 151
Starling's Law of the heart, 12
Stimuli for contraction, 17
Streptase, 146–147
Streptokinase (SK), 146–147
Strokes, reducing rate of, 146
Stroke volume, 11
Structure. *See* Cardiac anatomy
ST segment, 41, 54
ST segment depression, 55–56, 73, 121
    causes of, 55
    indicating lateral MIs, 113
    indicating posterior MIs, 123